## WHAT PROFESSIONALS ARE SAYING ABOUT *KANGAROO CARE*

"Given the powerful information within these covers, parents are empowered to practice the nurturing that is innate and a part of our cultural experience of being human. *Kangaroo Care* is a "must read" for expectant and newly delivered parents and health professionals that offer special infant care."

—Chandice Covington, Ph.D., R.N.C., P.N.P.
Wayne State University College of Nursing

"The authors have done a great and important job in researching and writing about Kangaroo Care."

—Elisabeth Bing, F.A.C.C.E.
author of *Six Practical Lessons for an Easier Childbirth*

"Kangaroo Care not only speeds and enhances the recovery of preterm infants, it can empower parents, reduce anxiety and strengthen the emotional and spiritual bond between parents and their babies."

—Vimala McClure
author of *Infant Massage: A Handbook for Loving Parents*
founder, International Association of Infant Massage Instructors

## WHAT MOTHERS ARE SAYING . . .

"During Kangaroo Care, I felt very calm and relaxed. It felt so comforting to have Cindy on my chest. It felt very natural. Besides the effect it was having on her, it was most therapeutic for me!"

"I feel more familiar with my baby now. I can handle her now without the fear of dropping or hurting her. I feel more at ease about positioning her to breastfeed. I'm even more excited about her coming home."

"It was so nice to be able to hold him and know that he likes to be held by his mommy. Just to be able to smell his hair—it was great!"

## AND FATHERS TOO!

"Much of my worry regarding my ability to handle him has dissipated. It was a very enjoyable experience, and I actually feel closer to him."

"This gave me so much joy. I have never felt so much happiness."

OTHER BOOKS BY SUSAN M. LUDINGTON-HOE
AND SUSAN K. GOLANT

*How to Have a Smarter Baby*


OTHER BOOKS BY SUSAN K. GOLANT

*No More Hysterectomies* with Vicki Hufnagel, M.D.

*Disciplining Your Preschooler and Feeling Good About It* with
Mitch Golant, Ph.D.

*Kindergarten: It Isn't What It Used to Be* with
Mitch Golant, Ph.D.

*The Joys and Challenges of Raising a Gifted Child*

*Getting Through to Your Kids* with Mitch Golant, Ph.D.

*Finding Time for Fathering* with Mitch Golant, Ph.D.

*Hardball for Women* with Pat Heim, Ph.D.

*50 Ways to Keep Your Child Safe*

*Taking Charge: Overcoming the Eight Fears of Chronic
Illness* with Irene Pollin, MSW (forthcoming)

# KANGAROO CARE

## The Best You Can Do to Help Your Preterm Infant

SUSAN M. LUDINGTON-HOE, CNM, PH.D.

AND

SUSAN K. GOLANT

BANTAM BOOKS
NEW YORK · TORONTO · LONDON · SYDNEY · AUCKLAND

Kangaroo Care
A Bantam Book/October 1993

Library of Congress Cataloging-in-Publication Data
Ludington-Hoe, Susan.
Kangaroo care : the best you can do to help your preterm infant / Susan
M. Ludington-Hoe and Susan K. Golant.
p.     cm.
Includes bibliographical references and index.
ISBN 0-553-37245-9
1. Infants (Premature)—Care.   2. Touch—Therapeutic use.
3. Parent and infant.   I. Golant, Susan K.   II. Title.
RJ250.L75     1993                        93-8485
618.92'011—dc20                            CIP

*Published simultaneously in the United States and Canada*

Bantam Books are published by Bantam Books, a division of Bantam
Doubleday Dell Publishing Group, Inc. Its trademark, consisting of the
words "Bantam Books" and the portrayal of a rooster, is Registered in
U.S. Patent and Trademark Office and in other countries. Marca
Registrada. Bantam Books, 1540 Broadway, New York, New York 10036.

PRINTED IN THE UNITED STATES OF AMERICA

FFG     0  9  8  7  6  5  4  3  2  1

*To*

*Mary Ellen Ludington Roach and Omid Seyed
Hashemi, whose constant skin-to-skin contact with me
when I was in intensive care made me survive when
no one thought it was possible.*


*And to the generations to come.*

# Contents

Lights  Inching into the Incubator  Graduating to the
Open-Air Crib  Transitions  Your Premie's Tumultuous
New World  Nursery Shutdown

## Contents

Helping Your Baby Regulate Her Temperature    Taking
Care of Yourself    Kangarooing Twins    What to Expect
After a Kangaroo Care Session    "Compliant Children"
Your Own Reactions

# Contents

# Foreword

Until recently, health professionals have discouraged parents from holding their preterm infants—the risk of harm and infection to these sensitive and fragile beings was too great.

Kangaroo Care, a program of skin-to-skin contact between parent and child, is part of the revolution in the care of premature infants. First researched in Latin America, Kangaroo Care was tested around the world during the 1980s, and it is quickly becoming a popular alternative for the treatment of premature infants. Neonatologists like myself are seeing great improvements in newborns who participate in Kangaroo Care. Not only do the sleeping and breathing patterns of premature infants improve, the babies appear to relax and become content from the touch of their parents' skin. Parents also benefit psychologically because they are allowed to play an active rather than a passive role in the recovery of their infant.

There is a need for high-technology intervention to help premature infants, but parents and babies are starving for one another's touch. As a neonatologist, I feel comfortable encouraging parents to use Kangaroo Care; it has been a positive experience for all of the babies (and parents) I have worked with and studied.

Susan Ludington-Hoe and Susan Golant have written a thorough, well-researched, and thoughtful guide to Kangaroo Care. The authors cover all aspects of the program—including its history, research basis, and practice—so that parents can make an informed choice to kangaroo their baby. I highly recommend this clear, step-by-step manual to any parent faced with the challenge of caring for a preterm infant.

—Anthony L. Hadeed, M.D.
Director, Neonatal Intensive Care Unit
Kadlec Medical Center

# Acknowledgments

Words of gratitude cannot fully express my appreciation of Dr. Gene Cranston Anderson, an inspiring nurse researcher and scholar—a mentor who has gently guided me past the turbulence encountered while forging a research career and directed me into a sea of scientific investigation while equipping me with the tools to meet the rigors of scientific inquiry. She is, in my mind and that of my colleagues, the Great Mother of Maternal-Newborn Mutual Caregiving nursing, and without her wisdom and support my research would not have been completed. She once related to me Louis Pasteur's adage "Chance favors the prepared mind" and I know that Dr. Anderson's mind opens worlds of opportunity for me and all of her other mentees. And I have benefited greatly as the bit of Prometheus living in my soul has tapped into Dr. Anderson's intellectual fire.

A clinical researcher depends upon the clinicians to perfect the possibilities of investigation, and to these fine nurses, Dottie Philips, Carol Thompson, Joan Swinth, Sudha Rao, Joanne Becker, Annie Hollingsead, Dr. Sharlene Simpson, Luz Angela Argote, Gladys Medellin, Lynnette Lippincott, and Teresa Warwood I am indebted, for making the studies feasible and the process fun. These nurses have volunteered countless hours for recruitment, data collection, and data reporting. As they become more involved, raising salient questions about Kangaroo Care and formulating methods to answer those questions, our work becomes stronger and they teach me so much. Two physicians need to be especially recognized for taking a chance on Kangaroo Care so that it could be validated and used with assurance. Kangaroo Care in the United States would be floundering without Dr. Anthony Hadeed, neo-natologist extraordinaire, who believes that mothers and babies belong together and is willing to challenge the status quo to carry through his philosophy. Similarly, Dr. Humberto Rey, Chair of Pediatrics for the Hospital Universitario del Valle in Cali, Colombia, took unprecedented steps when he let Kangaroo Care demonstrate its advantages and potential.

Without the babies and their mothers and fathers who have been the subjects in all the studies, there would be no Kanga-roo Care. The open-mindedness of all the parents and profes-sionals and countless other researchers who have been involved with Kangaroo Care will enable this important practice to endure.

I thank God for giving me a friend like Susie Golant, a writer who can capture my thoughts and express so eloquently the emotions and hopes surrounding this wonderful form of natural care-giving. And surely there is no other who tolerates my erratic schedule (or lack of schedule) as well.

And finally my gratitude to the staff of UCLA Medical Center Medical Intensive Care Unit is limitless for they are the *sine qua non* of this book. Thank you to all of you for helping me find ways to keep mothers and babies in touch with each other, together, forever.

Susan M. Ludington-Hoe


For my part, I would like to thank our editor at Bantam, Toni Burbank, who had the foresight and enthusiasm to get this project off the ground. Without her encouragement, this book would still be a gleam in Susan Ludington-Hoe's eye. I am grateful to Coleen O'Shea, whose insightful questions and comments helped us shape our work to best reach parents. And as always, I am indebted to our agent, Bob Tabian, who is ever watchful over our interests.

I'm also grateful to my husband, Mitch, who stands by me as an ally, friend, lover, cheerleader, and source of moral and material support. Without him, there are no books. And to my children, Cherie and Aimee, now almost fully grown, who have taught me about bonding and maternal love. Without them, there are no books. And to my parents, Arthur and Mary Kleinhandler, who nurtured, loved, and protected me. Without them, there is no me!

Finally, I'd like to thank Susan Ludington-Hoe for having the vision and the courage of her convictions. Through her generosity of spirit and inquiring mind, she has helped more families fall in love with their babies than anyone else I will ever know. For this and other gifts, I am grateful.

Susan Golant

# PART ONE

# What Is Kangaroo Care?

# 1

# Today's Revolution in Premature Care

A tiny premature baby was born 16 weeks early (24 weeks gestation) at Brigham and Women's Hospital in Boston, Massachusetts, in October 1991. Steven was quite sick, and the medical staff had great difficulty keeping him alive. It appeared that all the treatments they tried were ineffective. Sadly, Steven was slipping away: his blood values were dropping, and his immature lungs were unable to provide him with enough oxygen.

Under the direction of the nurses in the neonatal intensive care unit (the NICU), Steven was given to his mother, Dorothy, so she would have a chance to say good-bye. They left mother and baby alone and returned two hours later.

What a surprise awaited them upon their return! Dorothy was still holding Steven, who was still connected to all his equipment and monitors. But she had undressed him and had spontaneously placed him on her bare chest. When the nurse in charge took Steven's vital signs for what she thought was the last time, she noticed the level of oxygen in his blood had increased, the level of carbon dioxide had dropped (as one would want it to), his blood pressure was more stable, his breathing less labored.

The nurses contacted the resident, and together they asked

Dorothy to continue holding her baby throughout the night so that they could monitor his progress. Within twenty-four hours, Steven improved dramatically. When Dorothy grew tired, her husband Jack came in and took over holding their infant. Over the course of the next two days, Steven was continuously held in the intensive care nursery of this teaching hospital.

During those three days, Steven's physiological condition reversed. The health care staff continued doing everything possible to save his life. Dorothy and Jack were exhausted from their round-the-clock vigil, and the neonatologist suggested they reduce their holding to three hours a day. In the following weeks, they alternated evenings with each other, until Steven was taken out of the incubator and placed in an open-air crib. He was discharged from the hospital at four months of age. Several months later, Steven and his parents appeared on *Good Morning America*—a "miracle baby" and his family.

Heartened by this success, the health staff were eager to try holding with other premature infants. Soon babies whose breathing was regulated by ventilators were being placed on their parents' chests. By a happy accident, Dorothy and Steven had demonstrated the enormous benefits of Kangaroo Care.

## WHAT IS A PREMATURE BABY?

Despite the common belief that pregnancy lasts for nine months (36 weeks), ideally a full-term baby is born at 40 weeks. Any child born between 38 and 42 weeks is considered *full term*. Infants born in the thirty-seventh week of gestation or earlier are considered *premature* or *preterm*. We also call them *premies*.

Seven percent of all babies born in the United States are premature. That's about a quarter of a million babies a year. Although the number of preterm births has held steady for the last six years, today there are more premies than ever before in hospital neonatal intensive care units around the nation. Medical science has progressed to the point that physicians and nurses are now able to make efforts to save infants as early as 24 to 26 weeks gestational age (16 to 14 weeks early). As recently as 1986, such premature babies had little chance of survival.

Because technological advances help keep earlier and earlier deliveries alive with the increased likelihood of a quality life, many babies spend the first few weeks or months of their existence in hospital settings. One can expect a premie born at 26 weeks to be hospitalized for three months.

But hospitalization—so necessary for saving your premie's life—also has its drawbacks. All of a fetus's sensory systems are functioning, though not fully mature, from the eighteenth week of gestation. This means that from the moment of birth, your premie can see, feel, touch, smell, taste, and sense movement. In fact, his systems may be hypersensitive, because his brain is too immature to filter out unimportant messages. At the slightest noise, he may startle, his heart rate may increase, his breathing may stop, and he may turn from pink to blue. He squints to shut out the bright lights. And he quickly learns that touch is frequently followed by the pain of various medical treatments.

Despite his defenselessness, your baby must endure weeks or even months of vitally important yet invasive medical procedures in the high-tech isolation of the neonatal intensive care unit. Moreover, he is separated from you. In the NICU, health care personnel and machines monitor all of his bodily functions and you have limited opportunities to caress and cuddle him.

It is painful to see your infant's body covered with sensors and wires and tubes, to stand by helplessly and hear him wail as blood is drawn. It is frightening to learn that he has difficulty breathing or that he cannot maintain his body temperature without mechanical assistance. Machines, and not you, have become the controlling influence during the first few days or weeks of your child's life.

Confronted with such an experience, you may feel powerless to comfort him. Allowed only limited visits, you may struggle with fear, bewilderment, and longing, especially since you know that your premie, though very ill, is still a little person. He needs the warmth of your loving embrace and affection to recover, grow, and thrive.

## THE KANGAROO CARE REVOLUTION

Since 1983, however, there has been a revolution brewing in the treatment of premature babies. It is called Kangaroo Care, and it holds a dual promise: of helping preterm babies recover from the effects of their prematurity and of helping parents empower themselves and bond with their infants. Kangaroo Care—as a supplement to technical medical interventions— is simply the best you can do to help your premature infant. And it is a procedure that doesn't cost a penny—only parental love, cheerfully given.

During Kangaroo Care, hospital personnel will remove your diaper-clad baby from the incubator or crib and help you hold him upright, skin-to-skin and chest-to-chest. As your infant lies between your breasts for an hour or two, you will note that he calms down, snuggles in, and falls asleep. He may even try to nurse. Kangaroo Care puts a stop to the cacophony and confusion of events in the intensive care unit. It protects your child by allowing him to fall so deeply into slumber that nothing—no loud noises, no bright lights, not even heel sticks—may disturb him. Kangaroo Care is that simple, yet it provides untold benefits to both parents and infants.

## THE BENEFITS OF KANGAROO CARE

Why is it that Kangaroo Care can help premies recover from the effects of prematurity? Scores of international scientific studies have shown that Kangaroo Care offers the preterm infant many physical and emotional benefits. These include:

- A stable heart rate
- More regular breathing

- Improved dispersion of oxygen throughout the body
- Prevention of cold stress. (When a premie becomes too cold, he burns up much needed oxygen and calories to stay warm.)
- Longer periods of sleep (during which the brain matures)
- More rapid weight gain
- Reduction of purposeless activity which simply burns calories at the expense of the infant's growth and health
- Decreased crying
- Longer periods of alertness
- Opportunities to breastfeed and enjoy the healthful benefits of breastmilk
- Earlier bonding
- Increased likelihood of being discharged from the hospital sooner

In Chapter 6, "Why You Should Use Kangaroo Care," we will explore these benefits in greater detail.

The benefits to parents have also been documented. Those who have practiced Kangaroo Care feel more positive about the birth experience despite its inherent difficulty. They are eager and ready to bring their babies home, and feel confident in handling them because they have already enjoyed opportunities to bond with their infants and create a loving relationship. This is true of fathers as well as mothers. (See Chapter 2, "Kangaroo Care Promotes Bonding," and Chapter 12, "Especially for Dad.") In short, Kangaroo Care helps premature babies to recover as it enables their parents to lovingly, actively, and positively participate in their care.

## WHY KANGAROO CARE WORKS

How could such a simple, natural, low-tech form of care for high-tech babies be so effective and have so many medical benefits? It doesn't seem to make sense. Yet from research that

I and others around the world have been conducting, we know that it does happen. *Kangaroo Care cannot replace—but can supplement—the established medical strategies that correct breathing and other medical stresses premies experience.*

I believe that Kangaroo Care works so beautifully because of three factors affecting the infant:

- It creates conditions similar to those with which the premie had become familiar in utero, such as the proximity of the mother's heartbeat sounds and her voice coupled with the gentle rhythmic rocking of her breathing.
- It provides containment and allows for flexion (bending of the arms and legs).
- It protects the infant and offers him a reprieve from the stressful elements of the NICU.

I will explain these factors in greater detail in Chapter 7, "Why Kangaroo Care Works." But for the moment, bear in mind that Kangaroo Care is also a way in which you can actively assume your role as a parent and become part of your child's life and care as soon as it is medically safe to do so. Kangaroo Care speeds the desirable process of bonding with your preterm infant. For once you begin Kangaroo Care, you will soon see your baby's appreciation at being placed on your chest. His face and hands will relax, he'll stop flailing about, smile, and fall deeply asleep—activities that occur only when an infant feels safe, loved, and secure. And you will feel immensely relieved.

## CAN TWINS BE KANGAROOED?

Absolutely! If your twins are born prematurely, it is possible to hold them together (one on each breast), hold them separately (one at a time), or alternate with their father (holding one while he holds the other). In fact, one mother of twins held both infants on her chest for six hours. Both mother and babies slept and stayed warm! You'll find more about how to kangaroo twins and individual babies in Chapter 10, "Before, During, and After Kangaroo Care."

## WHAT IS THE PROOF THAT KANGAROO CARE WORKS?

When a procedure is this new, parents want to know what scientific evidence supports such favorable claims. I am happy to report that to date, over sixty research studies undertaken by numerous investigators have been published in scientific scholarly journals documenting the progress of thousands of premature babies in Kangaroo Care. Studies have been carried out in Scandinavia, England, France, Germany, India, Uganda, Kenya, Mozambique, throughout Central and South America, and in the United States.

The evidence is overwhelmingly positive. For example, many researchers have looked at breathing-ability patterns during Kangaroo Care and have found great improvements. Likewise, scientists have found improvements in weight gain, growth, motor development, relaxation, the likelihood of breastfeeding, and overall health and survival. The consensus is that in the long run, Kangaroo Care babies are doing well. The studies have been supported by countless clinical observations and reports.

Though this book concentrates on studies in the United States, these have evolved from groundbreaking research that began abroad. My own work was inspired by Dr. Gene Cranston Anderson, who introduced Kangaroo Care to the United States. (See Chapter 3, "The Birth of Kangaroo Care.")

UNICEF and the World Health Organization have already published documents recommending the use of Kangaroo Care. In addition to other ongoing research in the United States, the National Institutes of Health has given me a grant to continue investigating this field. When you read the evidence presented here, you will understand why I, among many other scientists and clinicians, am devoted to bringing this new form of caring and curing to as many premature babies as possible.

# A MOTHER'S STORY: MARY KANGAROOS BEN

Mary swung open the door to the now-familiar sights and sounds of the Neonatal Intensive Care Unit (NICU) at Kadlec Medical Center in Richland, Washington. Suddenly she was surrounded by a bustle of activity. Nurses moved deftly among the incubators and open warmers, tending to their tiny charges. Babies wailed that weak, high-pitched cry that only a premie can make; they were understandably discomforted at having their heels stuck with needles. All about, the clatter of metal instruments, the hum of x-ray machines, the glare of bright lights, and the tangle of wires—an electrician's nightmare— created a sense of ordered chaos. Mary was looking for her son. She had come for her daily visit with her new baby.

Ben was born two weeks earlier, at 30 weeks gestational age (10 weeks early). He required a ventilator to help him breathe for two days and had suffered from respiratory distress and infection. At birth, he weighed only 1,502 grams, about 3 pounds, 5 ounces.

Ben had been through a lot in his short life: He had had difficulty breathing, he couldn't eat or digest his food well, he slept fitfully and couldn't truly rest for any length of time. On his back, he seemed jittery under the unblinking watchfulness of bright warming lights. An octopus of wires emerged from Ben's small body; he was connected to monitors that constantly gauged the beating of his heart, his breathing, his oxygen levels, blood pressure, and temperature. As Ben was continually being poked, prodded, and evaluated in every way imaginable, it was no surprise he seemed irritable and uncomfortable.

Mary and her husband, Dave, had suffered as well. No sooner had Ben been born than they both became racked with questions and self-doubts. How could this have happened? they wondered. Did we do anything during the pregnancy to bring on premature labor? Why did this have to happen to us? To our first child? Will Ben survive? Will he have special needs once we bring him home? Their emotional wounds and fears ran deep.

But today Mary was to put these thoughts behind her. This was a big day. Ben was celebrating his second week birthday. But even more exciting, today Joan, the nurse attending this tiny infant, would show Mary how to provide him with Kangaroo Care.

As Mary entered the NICU, Joan flagged her down. "This way," she said as she escorted the young woman to a changing room. "Please take off your blouse and bra," Joan instructed, "and put on this yellow hospital gown with the opening to the front. Once you've changed, we'll get you comfortable beside Ben's incubator."

Mary changed quickly and found the stationary reclining chair set up next to Ben's incubator. She leaned over and noticed that in the bright lights and tumult of the intensive care unit, the boy seemed agitated: his arms and legs were flailing about.

Mary got comfortable and sat with her feet supported. Joan handed her the baby (who was wearing a diaper and a headcap) so that mother and son now were chest-to-chest, skin-to-skin. She positioned the baby's monitoring leads to make sure that they weren't tugging on him or making him uncomfortable. She placed Ben in a slightly diagonal, flexed position, with his knees tucked under his body to preserve heat and his head resting near Mary's left breast. For extra insulation, Joan folded a standard receiving blanket into fourths and put it across the baby's back. Then Mary closed the yellow hospital gown over Ben's covered body.

Immediately, Ben started to nuzzle in and relax. He decided to use his mother's left breast as a pillow. "Mary, you can talk, pat, and sing all you want until Ben falls asleep," Joan told her.

Mary followed Joan's cue. "That's great, sweetie," she cooed to her son. "Here, cuddle in. Are you warm and comfy? Don't worry. I have a good hold on you. You're such a good boy. Do you know how much I love you? But we'll talk later. Mommy wants you to get some sleep now. I'll bet you could use the rest."

Mary looked up at the nurse with a grateful smile, and tears glistened on her cheeks. Then she quietly gazed down at Ben

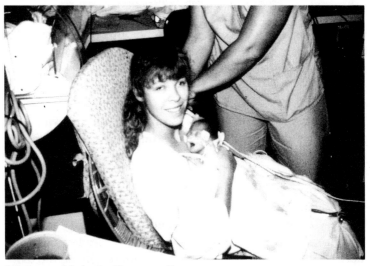
Mother and baby in Kangaroo Care

as he closed his eyes and relaxed his fingers. She sank back into the chair and began singing a lullaby.

Within a few minutes the infant drifted off to sleep. He remained there on his mother's chest, at peace, awakening only to suckle a bit. Mary was thrilled. She had wanted to breast-feed and had diligently pumped her breasts since Ben's birth, so she would be ready when the opportunity arose. And now, instinctively, Ben moved his head until he found her nipple. He opened his little mouth to get as much of the nipple as he could, but almost as soon as he had latched on, he drifted back to sleep.

Mary watched in wonder. She made sure that Ben's feet remained tucked under the blanket and then reclined a bit to make him and herself more comfortable. Soon, she too fell asleep. They remained together in peaceful slumber for two hours as the monitor alarms quieted: Ben's heart and breathing patterns had become more regular.

Suddenly Ben roused and started to cry. Mary awakened immediately to soothe him. "Are you hungry?" she asked, as she offered her left nipple in response to his slight mouthing movements and cries.

Joan noticed the activity. She came over and assisted them

by stabilizing Ben's head onto the breast and encouraging Mary's efforts to hold Ben in place while she depressed the breast tissue so Ben could breathe while sucking. The boy suckled for three minutes—a major accomplishment for a little premie's first breastfeeding experience.

After Ben had tired, Mary lifted him from her chest and placed him back in his incubator. Joan changed his diaper and laid him on his side within blanket boundaries, readjusting his monitor leads.

Mary was euphoric. "I've waited so long for this moment," she said, tears of joy streaming down her face. "It's such a relief to finally be close to my baby, to hold him and feed him and love him. Now, I really feel as though I'm his mother! He needs me. The days when I could only touch his little hand—they seemed like an eternity. Did you see? He even looked into my face. He really liked lying on my chest. I can't wait to tell Dave about this. He's going to come in to kangaroo Ben tomorrow. I feel like I can relax now. He's really ours."

The empowerment and the bonding that occurred as a result of Kangaroo Care were so potent that this mother, who had been deeply distressed by the problems engendered by her son's early arrival, gained the confidence that she needed to insure the safe passage of her infant from hospitalization to normal home care. Mary could now look forward to bringing her baby home with more comfort and self-assurance.

As you can see, the Kangaroo Care program is cheap, available, comforting, noninvasive, and easy. It will help you bridge time and deal with your infant's physical ills. What a magnificent gift from mother and father to baby.

# 2

# Kangaroo Care Promotes Bonding

Ginny became one of our Kangaroo Care parents at Kadlec Medical Center in Richland, Washington, when as part of a study, we asked her to come in to the NICU to hold her infant, Jesse, for a period of time on five consecutive days. Her experience demonstrates just how powerful a force bonding can be.

The first day of the experiment, Ginny approached the situation in a somewhat reserved way. She slipped into the NICU quietly, undressed in a shielded corner, and sat stiffly as the nurses positioned Jesse on her chest. On her pre–Kangaroo Care comment sheet she wrote, "I don't know if I should be doing this." Clearly she was anxious.

The second day, Ginny strode right into the room, got herself ready, and plopped into the recliner. She stretched out her arms to receive and help position her infant. On her post–Kangaroo Care comment sheet that day she wrote, "I really needed to do this."

On day three, Ginny nearly ran into the NICU, tearing off her T-shirt and throwing on the hospital gown as she approached her son's incubator. She sported a grin to rival the Cheshire Cat's as she lifted her son out of the incubator herself and placed him on her chest, positioning the wires down his side. On her comment sheet she wrote, "Kangaroo Care is the only thing for me! I enjoy it tremendously. I really, really, REALLY need to do this."

After day five, Ginny brought her husband along. As soon as they entered the nursery she turned to him and said, "Tom, I've got a surprise for you. Take your shirt off and scrub down." Then she led him to their son's incubator and said, "Now you get to hold the baby!"

Tom settled into the recliner, and he, too, began grinning as his wife positioned the little boy on his chest. Soon Tom was singing and rocking. Jesse smiled no less than five times during the thirty minutes that his dad held him.

Kangaroo Care gave the entire family the opportunity to bond—an opportunity that had been long in coming and sorely missed.

## WHAT IS BONDING?

During the first hour or two after birth, a healthy baby is calm and quiet. This is his first opportunity to look at his mother's face, recognize her voice, become familiar with her scent, adapt to her touch, seek out her breast, and snuggle down for a good meal and a nice nap. During this process, the infant begins bonding to his mother. With repeated experiences, bonding is cemented.

Bonding also involves a specific set of behaviors on the part of mothers as they lay claim to their newborns. It begins with a characteristic pattern of touch. When first introduced to her baby, a mother will begin exploring his cheeks and fingers with her fingertips. After about five or ten minutes, she will stroke him with the open palm of her hand and eventually engulf him in a loving embrace.

She'll begin talking to her baby, moving from the third person to the second and calling him by name: "Look at this baby. He's beautiful. Aren't you beautiful, Zachary?" She will express eagerness for her infant to make eye contact with her. "Won't you look at me, Zachary?" she'll ask. "I'm here. I'm your mommy."

Next, the mother will visually explore her baby, counting the toes and making sure that all the parts are working. She'll confirm the child's gender for herself. After the physical inventory, she'll start making comparisons and associations: "He's got my brother's nose and Aunt Sally's eyes. Look at those fingers. They're just like yours!" These associations are vital to helping a mother claim her baby. She knows he's hers; she has the right child.

Then, she'll ask the nurse or others about her newborn's characteristics. She'll ask about birthmarks, or about why the ears seem so soft. This stage is important, since the mother is becoming an advocate for her child.

Finally, when a mother refers to her infant as "my baby," or "my son," it becomes clear that bonding has begun. Fathers progress through the same stages when they visit and ultimately hold their babies.

## PREMATURE BIRTH ALTERS THE BONDING PROCESS

When a baby is born prematurely, bonding must often be deferred. When this happens, many parents worry that they have missed the opportunity to bond with their infants. Sharon, who had been released from the hospital earlier, approached me with this concern. She seemed almost frantic, and understandably so. "I just want to take Emily home and put her in bed with me and my husband," she sobbed. "I haven't been able to see her since she was born three days ago. I read about the bonding period being important the first few hours after birth. Dr. Ludington-Hoe, will this separation hurt my baby?"

Sharon's feelings were normal, and they trace back to events immediately following the delivery of a premature baby. Of necessity, the usual pattern must change. Your baby is taken away as soon as the umbilical cord is cut, and you are given no opportunity to touch or embrace her. Yet, at the moment of birth, that's what your body wants to do most! It nearly yells out, "Let me hold my baby!"

But in this critical situation, your premie is given to the

neonatal team of doctors and nurses immediately after birth. They clean her face, listen to her heart, blow oxygen by her nose and inflate her lungs, and, if necessary, place tubes down her throat for the ventilator. As they take these emergency measures, a team member may shout to you, "You have a baby girl," but you may only catch a brief glimpse of your newborn as the medical staff quickly carries her out to the intensive care unit.

Naturally, this causes you great anxiety. You haven't been allowed to see or hold your baby. Had you secured even two minutes with her, you would finally be able to visualize the child you had been imagining for so many months. You might have been able to reassure yourself that her eyes were open or that she possessed all the requisite fingers and toes. Yet sadly, in the present situation, you couldn't even hear her cry. The tubes in her throat prevented her from doing so.

Certainly, you may also experience tremendous fear for your infant's well-being. You worry if she will survive. In fact, your anxiety may redirect your focus from "this is my baby" to "will my child live?" Bonding, as important as it may be, gets placed on the back burner for now.

Besides, you can't simply jump off the delivery table and follow your infant into the intensive care nursery. Whether you've had a vaginal birth or a C-section, most likely your nurse-midwife or obstetrician will have to deal with the after-birth and sew up the episiotomy or incision. And if you send your baby's father to the nursery to see how the child is doing, you may feel even more distraught because you're now alone with your fears as well as coping with the very real emotional and physical aftereffects of labor and delivery.

## BONDING IN THE NICU

Be assured that a delay in holding and caressing your infant doesn't mean that bonding won't occur. In fact, you probably became psychologically attached to your baby before birth. Physical bonding certainly does occur, only a bit later. Bonding is not an all-or-nothing, I-have-to-do-this-in-the-first-two-hours-or-all-is-lost proposition. Even if the physical bonding process begins three days or two weeks after your child's birth, you will still go through it, although perhaps in a more fragmented manner.

As one Kangaroo Care mother put it, "All that stuff about bonding during the first two hours after birth is a bunch of hogwash! I couldn't love my baby any more than I do. In fact, I feel even more protective of him because he is a premie."

The process of bonding may not be as satisfying at first, however, since the technical equipment may prevent you from holding or even fully seeing your infant. Many parents are put

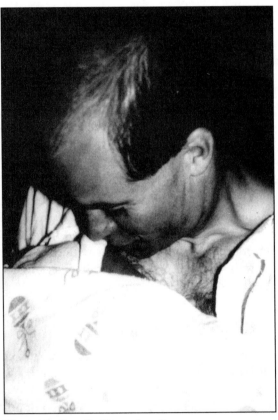

Kangaroo Care facilitates bonding.

off by all the tubes and wires entering and exiting their infant. They can't even see what he looks like because of them. I've found, though, that as parents learn what each tube and wire does, they are better able to ignore them and focus on their child.

Prepare yourself for your first visit with your premie in the NICU. You can say to yourself: "I know I'm going to be overwhelmed by all of the equipment. My goal on this first visit is just to see my baby's face. I probably won't get to see his eyes because they'll be closed. But I'll look at his pretty little lips. They'll be so small and delicate—almost like a porcelain figurine's. They'll be perfect but tiny."

It also helps to know that your premie won't be the picture of baby beauty—premature babies are not "Gerber babies"! One mother declared that her infant looked like a "skinned chicken"! Your infant's skin may be wrinkled and oddly colored, his ears unusually large and veined, and his head bald. But give him time! He will round out nicely in a few months; the fat that is usually added during the last four weeks of pregnancy will slowly but steadily get laid down as your newborn matures.

## BONDING DURING KANGAROO CARE

The chance to explore your baby's body with your fingertips and palm, to embrace and engulf him, to take an inventory, become acquainted, claim him as your own, and advocate for him—all this can come only with physical contact.

I believe it's hard to cement a connection until parent and baby have had the opportunity to touch. Even swaddling can interfere with this process. The sooner you can hold your infant in Kangaroo Care, the sooner you'll feel that warm, melting, loving sensation that comes with bonding, and the sooner you can reassure yourself that you and your infant have established an affectionate relationship.

As you embrace your child, you're able to touch him and look at him. I have seen mothers change visibly at this point. Their faces and bodies relax. They smile. At first, they may look around the room, but soon they refocus and concentrate only on their infants. You, too, may find that Kangaroo Care relieves you of some of your anxiety. As one mother put it, "I know I need to hold my baby next to me. It calms me down and helps me cope with all the NICU procedures."

## HOW KANGAROO CARE REDUCES PARENTS' ANXIETY

Researchers have found that four factors make parents really anxious in the NICU.

1. *The sights and sounds of intensive care.* Parents and babies alike are surrounded by constant noise and activity. Beeping alarms, crying infants, bustling technicians, and other distressed parents are all upsetting.

2. *The behavior and communication patterns of the staff.* You may find that nurses and doctors don't have the time to explain what they're doing in adequate detail. They may go over procedures too quickly or use words you don't understand. Receiving seemingly conflicting information about your child (e.g., one nurse telling you that your infant is doing well while another says that she had to increase his oxygen level by 5 percent) can be especially disturbing.

If you find yourself feeling frustrated, don't hesitate to let the nurses know that you need them to take five minutes to go over all of the information they have imparted in the last few days. They may need to repeat certain information two or three times (and explain it in different ways, drawing pictures if necessary) before you fully understand it. Nurses excel in educating parents and that is part of their practice.

3. *Your baby's behavior and appearance.* The equipment used for your child may be intimidating, and perhaps more worrisome is your infant's unusual color (pale or jaundiced), uneven breathing, small size, wrinkled appearance, jerky restlessness, or limpness. If your baby looks sad or afraid or if he cries, that can exacerbate your concern.

4. *Your lack of a relationship with your infant.* The physical separation, your inability to feed or hold your child when you want to, the lack of privacy, and your powerlessness to protect

your infant from pain and painful procedures can heighten your anxiety. Many parents of premies feel helpless about intervening on their babies' behalf.

I have observed and measured all of these factors in mothers before they started Kangaroo Care and after they experienced the procedure for a three-hour one-time visit and for 10 to 15 hours spread out over five consecutive days. I am happy to report that after Kangaroo Care, mothers report feeling much less anxious about their babies' appearance and behavior and about being unable to create a relationship. And so, not only does Kangaroo Care give a mother the opportunity to hold her baby so that she can go through the process of bonding, but it also seems to reduce the anxiety and stress that could inhibit the process.

## THE SHORT- AND LONG-TERM BENEFITS FOR PARENTS

Dr. Dyanne Affonso, a professor of family health nursing at the University of California, San Francisco Medical Center, studied the short- and long-term benefits Kangaroo Care has for par-

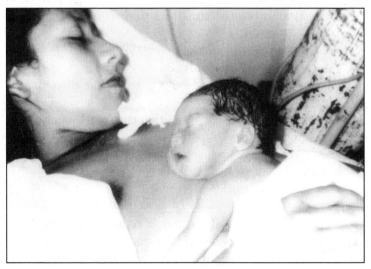

A mother and baby at peace during Kangaroo Care.

ents. She found that Kangaroo Care mothers whose babies were still hospitalized expressed confidence in their ability to breastfeed and care for their infants; they were comfortable in the nursery and eager for discharge. The non-kangarooing mothers in her study frequently abandoned breastfeeding, felt anxious in the nursery, and were hesitant about taking their babies home.

When Dr. Affonso interviewed these same women two years after the birth of their children, she found a similar pattern. The mothers who had provided Kangaroo Care had gotten "closure" over the experience. During their interviews, they talked about their baby's future and how well their baby was doing. They often expressed the feeling that they had done the best they could.

Unfortunately, the mothers not involved in Kangaroo Care had not resolved their issues relating to the premature birth. They were still asking themselves, "Why me?" "Why this baby?" "What could I have done better?" And they were still trying to resolve their grief and guilt. They had not yet fully come to terms with the premature birth.

My observations bear out Dr. Affonso's research. Parents in my studies who have an opportunity to experience Kangaroo Care have similar positive responses to their infants. In addition:

- They feel close to their infants.
- They express confidence about monitoring their babies' health.
- They feel that "it's about time" that they're allowed to have this contact.
- They start to have a sense of confidence that their baby is well cared for and may survive.
- They feel in control.

As one mother who had previously expressed anxiety about being able to care for her infant once she got her home observed after her Kangaroo Care experience, "I feel more familiar with my baby now. I'm able to understand her cries a little better. I can handle her now without the fear of dropping or hurting her. I feel more at ease about positioning her to breastfeed. I'm even more excited about her coming home."

Kangaroo Care can reduce stress in mothers as well as babies. As another mother explained after her session, "During Kangaroo Care, I felt very calm and relaxed. It felt so comforting for me to have Evelyn on my chest. It felt very natural. Besides the effect it was having on her, it was therapeutic for me! Having that skin-to-skin contact was heaven. All my worries and apprehensions toward her were immediately alleviated. I am *sure* any mother participating in Kangaroo Care will be greatly rewarded."

Kangaroo Care is empowering. When a mother experiences this form of loving touch, she knows that she is doing something special for her infant that no one else can do. She senses that her baby recognizes her. She sees that he is relaxed and in deep sleep. Kangaroo Care can provide positive closure for what has been a difficult, traumatic experience.

As yet another mother explained, "It was so nice to be able to hold him and know that he likes to be held by his mommy. Just to be able to smell his hair—it was great!" Kangaroo Care is healing to baby and parents alike.

# 3

# The Birth of
# Kangaroo Care

It seems unlikely that in our society, with its emphasis on high-tech medicine, doctors and nurses would willingly remove preterm infants from the carefully monitored and machine-generated warmth of their incubators and place them on their mother's chests. Indeed, Kangaroo Care originated not in the United States but in Bogota, Colombia, where in 1983 two neonatologists, Dr. Edgar Rey and Dr. Hector Martínez, reported on a dramatic treatment designed to save preterm babies.

The mortality rate for premies in Colombia was 70 percent. (By contrast, the mortality for very low birthweight babies [3 pounds] in the United States was 39 percent and for 3- to 5-pound babies was only 3 percent.) Colombian premies were dying of infections and respiratory problems. Even today, most of Colombia's public hospitals have few working incubators, no sterile formula, and few room heaters. Electric power is inefficient and unreliable. Equipment, if it exists at all, is likely to be aged or broken. When an incubator does function, several babies must share it, thus dramatically increasing the potential for infection.

In addition, according to the Colombian minister of health, mothers who gave birth to preterm infants often resisted becoming bonded and attached to them, because they believed the infants would not survive these harsh circumstances. Some premies died from lack of attention and failure-to-thrive syndrome. Others were simply abandoned.

The hospital in Bogota at which Drs. Rey and Martínez practiced had no heat. That city is on a high plain in the Andes. The climate is relatively cold, the average temperature being around 50° Fahrenheit.

Drs. Rey and Martínez realized that medical conditions were less than optimal for saving premies. Having little hope that the situation would quickly change, they decided to give the babies to their mothers to hold in skin-to-skin contact. Perhaps, the neonatologists speculated, more could be done by the women themselves than with the meager assistance the medical establishment could provide. The babies would have quick, easy, and on-demand access to their mother's breasts for feeding. That would help them gain weight and provide immunity to the infections to which prematures are so prone. The babies would also be kept warm. Drs. Rey and Martínez felt they had everything to gain and nothing to lose.

These neonatologists instructed the mothers of the premies under their care to hold their babies 24 hours a day. The women were to sleep with their babies and carry them everywhere they went. They literally "wore" their babies under their blouses, tucked into their brassieres, or supported by knotted shawls forming pouches—hence the name "Kangaroo Care."

The experiment worked. Drs. Rey and Martínez noted a precipitous drop in neonatal mortality with these premies—from 70 to 30 percent. Importantly, the use of Kangaroo Care decreased the likelihood that mothers would abandon their premies. The babies were gaining weight and surviving, and the mothers were becoming attached to their infants.

When these two physicians presented their findings at an international meeting, the First Course of Fetal and Neonatal Medicine at the Instituto Maternal-Infantil in Bogota, they attracted worldwide interest and the involvement of the World Health Organization and UNICEF. The Swedes,

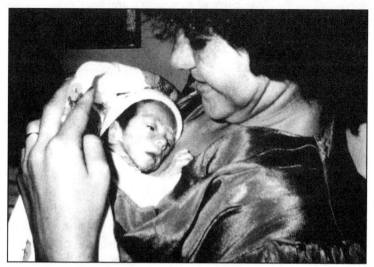

A baby in Kangaroo Care peeking out from his mother's blouse.

Dutch, and British were quick to utilize Kangaroo Care in their neonatal hospital settings and to start scientific evaluations of its usefulness. From 1983 to 1986, European scientists were investigating the benefits of Kangaroo Care but no one was yet practicing or researching it in the United States.

## HOW I BECAME INVOLVED

I first heard about Kangaroo Care in 1986 at the biennial meeting of the International Congress of Infant Studies. There Dr. Gene Cranston Anderson, Professor of Nursing at the University of Florida in Gainesville, presented a video demonstrating the technique she had seen in a visit to Drs. Rey and Martínez in Bogota.

The film showed a Colombian mother bringing her kangarooing premie, then 38 weeks postconception, back to the hospital for a daily checkup. The young woman came into the clinic wearing her baby under her clothes, his little head emerging from the collar of her blouse. The infant was weighed and measured and returned to his position on his mother's chest, where he seemed perfectly contented and relaxed.

I was mesmerized by the film, not simply because it broke new ground (which it did) but because this young woman continuously stroked her baby's head. It seemed to me that at least some of the baby's relaxation and contentment was a reflection of this repetitive caressing. I believed that the benefits ascribed to Kangaroo Care might have been, in part at least, a function of the loving touch I had observed. I was particularly interested in the effects of touch because years earlier, for my doctoral research at Texas Women's University and postdoctoral research at Baylor University, I had investigated how rhythmic, repetitive stroking helped infants gain weight soon after birth.

As I watched Dr. Anderson's Kangaroo Care video my mind jumped back to the babies I had studied earlier. The Colombian premie exhibited the same deep relaxation that I had observed in my stroking studies. Dr. Anderson explained that Kangaroo Care babies were responding to their environment in a peaceful, non-stressed way. They were also gaining weight better than those who were not in Kangaroo Care. I then speculated that the stroking was playing a part.

In 1987, I had an opportunity to observe Kangaroo Care for myself. Because of my research and writings on infant development and infant stimulation (*How to Have a Smarter Baby* with Susan K. Golant, Bantam, 1986), the Colombian Ministry of Health called upon me to consult on ways to minimize the abandonment of preterm babies and to enhance attachment for all children.

This invitation arrived simultaneously with an inquiry from EMESFAO, the Colombian Society for Psychoprophylaxis in Obstetrics and Gynecology. This group of physicians and nurses asked me to come to Bogota to share new approaches to fetal stimulation. They wanted to know what mothers could do during pregnancy to enhance maternal bonding.

I replied to both groups that I would be delighted to come if they would teach me something in return. I wanted to learn about Kangaroo Care. Happily, Dr. Anderson secured permission to investigate Kangaroo Care at the Instituto Maternal-Infantil, the main referral hospital for high-risk babies in Bogota.

Unfortunately, we were unable to complete the study Dr. Anderson had planned, because economic difficulties had forced the hospital to refuse new patients during the weeks of our visit. We did, however, get to see mothers practicing Kangaroo Care with hospitalized babies who were nearing discharge from the intensive care nursery and others who had already been discharged and were making regular visits to a follow-up clinic called La Casita (built by the World Health Organization in response to Drs. Rey and Martínez's work).

In the hospital, the mothers came to the special breastfeeding room adjacent to the nursery where physicians positioned the babies on their chests. Mothers sat with their infants in Kangaroo Care for several hours. During this time, they waited for their babies to smell their breastmilk, move toward the breast, root, latch on, and suck. If the babies were able to coordinate sucking, swallowing, and breathing, nurses allowed the mothers to go home with their infants in Kangaroo Care, with instructions to return the very next day, when checks for weight gain and signs of infection would be made.

If a returning baby had not gained weight, nurses gave him his mother's expressed breastmilk through a small tube down the throat into the stomach while the mother held him in Kangaroo Care. Mothers could come back daily for free follow-ups. (The World Health Organization picked up the tab.) Eventually, as the babies got stronger, they came every other day, then once a week, twice a month, and so on until the infants were at least a year old.

Ironically, during our three-week stay in Bogota, I observed no stroking. Not a single mother participating in the Kangaroo Care project stroked her baby the way that woman had on the video, yet the infants were certainly just as contented and relaxed without it. Not only that, they were gaining weight beautifully and staying well. All of this said to me that I should look into this phenomenon further. It seemed clear to me that Kangaroo Care was a different form of touch—not the rhythmic, intermittent stroking I had previously investigated but a continuous, embracing, containing form of touch, perhaps much like what the infant might have experienced in utero.

Unable to obtain any research data in Colombia, I sought out clinical sites to test Kangaroo Care in the United States. This was no easy task. The idea of having parents take their premature babies out of incubators and hold them on their chests was foreign to many of the professionals sitting on the review boards that must approve human experimentation studies.

After approaching and being turned down by eight hospitals, I finally found, at Hollywood Presbyterian Medical Center in Los Angeles, a neonatologist who believed so strongly in the importance of human contact for health—even beginning in the premature nursery—that he would help get a study approved. Together, Dr. Anthony Hadeed and I approached yet another review board, and in 1988 we succeeded in getting approval to test Kangaroo Care with babies who were getting ready to go home from the intensive care nursery.

And so, in 1988 I began researching Kangaroo Care in the United States. Starting in California, my research expanded along the West Coast and then, in 1991, to international sites as well.

One of my first and perhaps most fascinating findings was that mothers unconsciously regulate their premies' skin temperatures by changing their own temperature in response. When we monitored the skin temperature of mothers' breasts, we found that it increased when their premies began to cool, and dropped when their babies warmed up.

After observing this phenomenon with twelve mother-infant pairs, my research associates Carol Thompson, Joan Swinth, and I wondered if *telling* a woman that her infant was becoming cold would hasten her regulating her own temperature. We decided to give it a try. Standing behind a mother, Carol told her, "Looks like your baby is becoming a little cold." Within two minutes, her breast temperature shot up two full degrees centigrade (about 3.6° Fahrenheit). That brought the premie's skin temperature up.

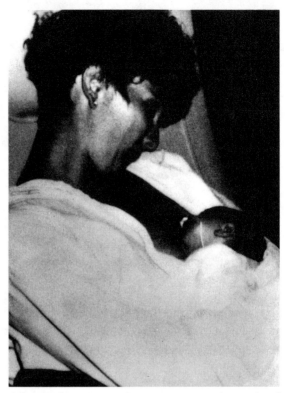

A baby's skin temperature is unconsciously regulated by the mother's skin temperature during Kangaroo Care.

Once the baby's skin temperature approached the upper limit, I told this mother, "He's warm enough now." And sure enough, over the next two minutes, her breast temperature fluctuated one to two degrees centigrade to keep the baby at a steady, normal temperature. We call this unconscious regulation "maternal-neonatal thermal synchrony." This discovery of a biological and behavioral dance between mother and baby is not dissimilar to other researchers' findings that infants move in time to maternal speech.

Our research yielded many other fascinating discoveries, and I'll share them with you throughout this book. But first, let's look at what your preterm infant must contend with immediately after birth and while in the intensive care unit.

# 4

# Life in the Neonatal Intensive Care Unit

To understand why Kangaroo Care is so beneficial, it's useful to retrace a premie's typical stay in the intensive care unit. The following scenario conveys the high-tech, somewhat impersonal clinical care with which a premie is bombarded upon birth. It describes the stages your infant might go through. This chapter will also help you understand the jargon and machinery in the intensive care unit.

We'll look at baby Nancy's case, since it's fully representative of a premie's difficult entry into the world.

## AN EARLY ARRIVAL

Nancy was born at 30 weeks gestational age—10 weeks early. At first, her parents, Allison and Jerry, had anticipated a "normal" birth. They had eagerly awaited their Lamaze classes and had hoped to deliver their child in a Labor-Delivery-Recovery-Postpartum room, a homelike environment in which they could stay together. Like so many other parents, they imagined that their baby would be placed in their loving arms soon after birth. They fantasized that they would be exhausted but would experience a sense of completion, wholeness, and awe at the miracle they had created.

Unfortunately, that was not to be the case. Labor began at the twenty-sixth week of pregnancy, forcing Allison to remain in bed. But despite bed rest, medication, and eventually even hospitalization, the contractions continued unabated. By 30 weeks Allison's cervix had dilated to more than 4 centimeters. In order to spare herself and her baby severe infection, Allison and Jerry decided with the advice of their obstetrician to deliver the baby 10 weeks early by C-section. (A vaginal birth was deemed too risky, since it could batter the premature infant's delicate skull.)

Rather than the lovely birthing environment they had envisioned, Allison was wheeled into a sterile operating room to deliver. Rather than holding their firstborn infant immediately after birth, she saw her baby whisked away from them as soon as she emerged from her mother's body—standard procedure in all premature births.

## THE MEDICAL TEAM WORKS ON A PREMIE

Upon delivery, the obstetrician immediately handed Nancy to the *neonatologist* (a physician specializing in newborns), who rushed her to the resuscitation bed in the delivery room. There several people worked on her at once: Linda, the neonatal nurse-practitioner, dried her off, while the neonatologist assessed her breathing and heart rate.

Nancy was able to draw a breath, but it was quite shallow and her cry was weak. Her pink color began to fade, and she became pale. The staff blew oxygen by her face to stimulate her respirations.

Nancy heaved again, took in a little more air and, as we say in the delivery room, "pinked up" but was unable to sustain this effort. Soon each breath was accompanied by grunts of increasing intensity. The labored breathing was audible even without a stethoscope, and as the staff watched Nancy's chest, they saw that, with each inhalation, the tissue was sucked in around her ribs and neck. Nancy flared her nostrils as if to gather in as much air as she possibly could. It was obvious that she was having a difficult time maintaining her breathing.

Meanwhile, Allison's incision was being sewn up, a procedure that took forty-five minutes. She had been fully awake, though anesthetized from the sternum down, during the C-section and had listened to the doctors as they delivered her baby. Sitting at the head of the operating table, Jerry described what he could see from behind the surgical drape. When the doctors rushed Nancy to the resuscitation bed, Jerry followed them. He stood back but watched what was going on, reporting to Allison from time to time. "They're drying her off now," he said. And then, "She looks pale. They're giving her oxygen."

At this point, the anesthesiologist gave Allison a sedative to relax her, and eventually she was wheeled into the recovery room, where she would stay for two hours. The nurses there checked her heart, oxygen levels, and ability to move as she came out of the anesthesia. When she awakened adequately, she was sent to a hospital room with IVs for antibiotics, fluids, and patient-controlled painkiller.

But Jerry stayed behind. Concerned by the activity surrounding his daughter, he stayed by the resuscitation bed to watch over her.

## SO MANY TUBES AND WIRES

Linda, the neonatal nurse-practitioner, put a tube down Nancy's throat and into her lungs to insure that the newborn was receiving adequate oxygen. And so Nancy was *intubated*. This tube was connected to a machine (a *ventilator*, also known as a *respirator*) that provided a specific level, volume, and pressure of oxygen—to keep her lungs open and give her the oxygen she needed.

Once the tube was inserted and Nancy's breathing became relatively stable, she was hurried to the intensive care nursery and placed on an open flat bed that had a warming unit (called a *radiant warmer*) directly above. At this point, the neonatologist allowed Linda and the intensive care nursery staff to take over.

Linda taped to Nancy's belly a small metallic disk (called a *servo-control*) that communicated her body temperature to the warming unit. This apparatus reacts automatically to any changes in the infant's temperature. Should it drop, the unit emits more heat to keep her warm. In this way, Nancy uses her precious oxygen and calories for recuperation and growth rather than to maintain her temperature.

Immediately Linda inserted an intravenous line into Nancy's scalp to provide fluid, as she expected Nancy to lose a lot of body fluid under the warmer. She also put a little tube into her umbilical cord (an *umbilical artery catheter*) to enable the intensive care nurses to measure the internal blood pressure, blood flow, and blood oxygen levels, and to get blood samples without having to repeatedly stick the infant with needles.

Then Linda started Nancy on an IV at the crook of the elbow, threading the tube through the vein in her arm, up to the heart (a *percutaneous line*). Through this tube, the nurses would provide the nutritional fluid called *parenteral nutrition*. This nutrition is introduced directly into the blood because that's more efficient than sending it to the stomach first.

Each tube and wire was then connected to its own pump or irrigation line. That's why the nurses had Nancy in an open bed: They could reach all of their equipment, move it in response to her movements, make changes minute-by-minute, and keep the machinery operational without having to fuss with the portholes on an enclosed incubator.

Next, Linda attached electrode leads and wires under each arm and on one leg. These connected to a monitor which displayed Nancy's heart rate and respiratory rate.

The staff had been continuously monitoring Nancy's *oxygen saturation*. You'll hear this referred to as $SaO_2$ or $O_2Sat$ in conversation in the intensive care nursery. An infant's oxygen saturation means how much oxygen the blood is carrying. Each hemoglobin molecule (the portion of the blood cell that carries the oxygen) is supposed to contain four oxygen molecules for 100 percent oxygen saturation. We try to keep the level between 92 and 97, if the infant needs oxygen assistance. Nancy's $O_2$ Sat was quite low at birth—78. But as the staff continued watching the monitor, it rose to 94.

Oxygen saturation is measured by a tiny dual sensor (a *pulse oximeter*) placed over the infant's skin on the finger, toe, earlobe, side of the foot, or palm. One sensor sends a tiny laser beam to the other, enabling the mechanism to determine if the hemoglobin cells are carrying the proper number of oxygen molecules.

Each heartbeat makes the vessels through which the oxygenated blood flows swell. During this pulse the sensor picks up the saturation level and tells us how much oxygen is actually getting to the tips of the infant's fingers and toes.

## UNDER THE WARMING LIGHTS

Nancy was all hooked up. The staff was now able to monitor her progress and determine how often the ventilator would breathe for her. They would make every effort to keep her respiration, oxygen, temperature, and blood volume and pressure within the normal range and provide the fluids and nutrients she needed to compensate for the fluid and weight loss she would experience under the radiant warmer. In addition, Linda wrote the orders for medications to regularize Nancy's breathing (*theophylline*) and help her lungs mature (*betamethasone*).

Over the course of the next five days, however, all did not go perfectly. Like so many premies, Nancy began showing signs of infection: irritability, high temperature, and a rapid heart rate (*tachycardia*). The intensive care nurse had to change the ventilator settings to make sure Nancy got enough oxygen but not too much. Nancy always had a nurse by her side. For 24 hours a day, the nurses gave Nancy intravenous antibiotics and adjusted her feedings, because in her sick state, she had to be fed slowly and continuously through the percutaneous line.

But eventually Nancy began to improve. As she recovered from the infection, she still had some breathing problems, but she didn't need as much oxygen as she had at first nor did she need the same amount of oxygen pressure. The nurses changed the ventilator setting to *CPAP* (*continuous positive airway pressure*). Rather than taking great big breaths in and out for the baby, the machine now maintained a small amount of constant pressure to keep the airway open. Similarly, the antibiot dosages were reduced, and eventually Nancy no longer needed them.

Soon the staff noticed that Nancy was beginning to make a spontaneous effort to breathe by herself. Instead of the respirator breathing every breath for her, it was set to breathe four out of five breaths. As she grew stronger each day, they were able to reduce this even further. Every once in a while, however, Nancy would forget to breathe (these breathing lapses are called *apnea*). In those instances, the nurse touched her body or called her name to provide the stimulation to bring on the breathing pattern again.

Simultaneously, Nancy began opening and closing her mouth deliberately, but not sucking. Instead of losing weight, as she had at first, she now began to gain weight. The nurses slowly cut back on the amount of nutrition going into the vein and supplemented her parenteral feedings with breastmilk which Allison had been pumping and saving for her baby. The nurses put a special nipple into Nancy's mouth and threaded a tube through it and down her throat. For one feeding a day the nurses were able to deliver some of Allison's breastmilk directly into Nancy's stomach. (This tube feeding is called *gavage feeding*. Mother's milk or fortified formula can be used.) The nipple helped to teach Nancy to associate the good feeling of fullness with sucking.

Three hours after her first "meal," the nurses measured how much milk remained in Nancy's stomach by reinserting a tube, this time attached to a syringe. When they drew back on the syringe, they could measure how much milk Nancy was able to digest and what was left over. If more than 5 cubic centimeters (about one-sixth of an ounce) remained (this is called the *residual*), that would signal that she was not digesting as well as the staff would have liked and consequently was unable to handle the same amount of milk in the next gavage feeding.

Another way to obtain this information is for the nurse to measure the infant's abdominal circumference. If that is becoming enlarged, it means the infant is distended with the food and not digesting, and therefore still too immature to handle an increase in quantity.

Fortunately, Nancy was ready for the milk. Over time she could take an adequate number of calories from the gavage tube. The staff was able to remove the percutaneous line, and Nancy graduated to the status of a *gavage-fed* baby. In fact, whenever Allison was available, we put Nancy to her breast, even with the tube down her throat, so that mother and baby could begin getting the hang of breastfeeding. (See Chapter 11, "Breastfeeding During Kangaroo Care.")

At 33 weeks postconception, Nancy started demonstrating strong sucking movements. The next time Allison visited, the staff weighed the infant and then asked Allison to put her to the breast without the gavage tube. After the feeding, they weighed Nancy again. Since she hadn't taken in enough milk, they asked Allison to express some fresh breastmilk into a miniature bottle fitted with a special premature-sized nipple. This nipple, called a *premie nipple*, is designed much like the human breast. It prevents flooding of the mouth, which impairs the developing coordination of sucking and swallowing and can cause choking. It also helps the baby build the strength of the 50 muscle bands around her mouth used for sucking.

The nurses alternated gavage feeding with nipple feeding. As you might expect, they gradually decreased the number of gavage feedings and soon let Nancy become solely nipple fed. Since Nancy began to take nutrition by sucking, we called her a *nippling baby*.

## INCHING INTO THE INCUBATOR

The transition from gavage to nipple feeding usually occurs when a baby is in an incubator. Much to the staff's and her parents' delight, this little girl was getting better; she was eating more and gaining weight.

The nurses moved Nancy into an incubator when she was able to breathe spontaneously. Her lungs inflated sufficiently to bring in oxygen and deflated without collapsing. With these positive signs and good oxygen saturation, they took Nancy off the ventilator and put two little oxygen-emitting prongs (*cannula*) up her nose to provide a higher concentration of oxygen.

The nurses watched the oxygen saturation levels while Nancy was on the cannula. Over the course of a few days, they felt it safe to decrease the amount of oxygen, and when Nancy was able to maintain oxygen saturation of 92 to 97 percent, they removed the cannula to observe how well she did on room air. Because her breathing appeared a little labored in room air, they put her in a little oxygen hood and added oxygen when she needed it (especially when being fed or moved). *Blow-by oxygen* can also be used at this point: An oxygen-emitting tube is placed by the infant's nose, so that a higher concentration of oxygen literally blows by the infant's nose.

As often occurs at this stage, the nurses found that they could reduce the medicine Nancy needed to control her breathing and help her lungs mature. They started weaning her from these medicines, but as they did, they watched carefully for breathing setbacks. It's not uncommon for babies to need time to adjust to cutbacks in their medication. Some begin having periods of apnea once off the drugs and must be put right back on them. In that case, we must wait a few days and try again. During the adjustment period as we reduce the medication, babies may need more frequent reminders to breathe (the nurses gently rub their skin when the apnea monitor sounds) and modifications in their medicine dosages.

In most cases, I recommend waiting to start Kangaroo Care until after the ventilator tube has been removed because it's harder to position an infant properly with the tube in place. (See page 116.) In this case the nurses took Nancy out of the incubator so her parents could begin to hold and cuddle her skin-to-skin. Allison and Jerry were eager to start Kangaroo Care. They had grown weary of trying to touch their infant by poking their fingers through an incubator porthole. What a pleasure it was for them to finally achieve their dream of being a loving family together.

## GRADUATING TO THE OPEN-AIR CRIB

While Nancy was in the incubator, the nurses still regulated her temperature using the servo-control, but when they wanted to see how she would adjust to being outside the incubator, they swaddled her in two receiving blankets and put her into an open-air crib. Then they checked her underarm temperature every three hours. As long as it remained over 36.7° centigrade (98° Fahrenheit), they allowed her to stay in the crib. They observed Nancy for 48 hours to determine whether her temperature stabilized.

They considered leaving Nancy in an open-air crib when she demonstrated that:

- She could be out of the incubator without any drop in temperature.
- She could gain weight consistently at the rate of 10 to 20 grams ($^1/_3$ to $^2/_3$ ounce) per day.
- She had been weaned from her oxygen needs and from medications such as theophylline, betamethasone, and antibiotics.
- Her breathing pattern and heart rate had stabilized.

Before going home, most premies remain in open-air cribs from 12 hours to five days depending on room availability, hospital practice, and the infant's condition. Nancy stayed for four days.

In the open-air crib, Nancy's main responsibilities were to continue to gain weight while breathing normal concentrations of oxygen and to maintain a normal breathing pattern while being fed. At this stage, the nurses asked Allison to come in daily to dress, feed, change, and move her baby around, in much the same way that she would at home. Although Nancy required no take-home equipment, other premies might. So, at this point parents may also learn which monitors (such as a home apnea monitor) may accompany their baby home and how to respond if an alarm sounds.

Once Nancy had shown that she had normal breathing, heart rate, weight gain, and adaptation to the movements and stimulations that confronted her in the open-air crib, she was deemed ready to go home. She had attained the ripe old age of 34 weeks 4 days postconception. Now the nurses asked Allison to spend Nancy's last 24 hours of hospitalization with her. Allison slept at the hospital, taking over feedings, diaper changes, bathing, and other child-care duties with the support of the nursing staff.

And so, less than five weeks after Nancy's somewhat traumatic birth, Allison and Jerry were able to take their baby home, knowing that they now had the loving tools to care for her.

## TRANSITIONS

In general, premies progress from continual to intermittent monitoring and from internal to external monitoring. Let's trace these transitions in greater detail.

**Monitoring.** When Nancy was born, we inserted many catheters into her body to monitor its internal changes. As she improved, we removed these internal lines but continued to monitor her condition by placing probes on her skin. As she progressed even further and moved into an open-air crib, we eliminated all of the monitoring equipment and performed intermittent evaluations every two to three hours. Some hospitals continue monitoring until the infant is discharged.

**Medical Access.** Nancy moved from an open radiant warmer tray to an incubator to an open-air crib to home. At first she had constant one-to-one attention. Eventually, she was able to share one nurse with three other babies.

**Breathing.** Nancy proceeded from a ventilator to continuous positive airway pressure (CPAP) to oxygen by cannulas to an oxygen hood to room air.

**Oxygen Saturation.** Room air is only 21 percent oxygen. At first, the nurses provided Nancy with a high concentration of oxygen because her immature lungs were inefficient at picking up oxygen that was available in room air: 90 to 95 percent of the air she breathed through the respirator was pure oxygen. After she recovered from her infection, they began turning down the oxygen concentration as they vigilantly monitored the oxygen saturation in her blood. As long as the saturation was good (92–97 percent), the weaning process continued over the course of many days. Eventually she needed only a 25 to 28 percent concentration of the gas to maintain good saturation. At that point, they turned off the oxygen and observed how she did on room air.

Toward the end of her hospitalization, Nancy was able to maintain a good saturation level without extra oxygen. She was continually pink and had no trouble breathing room air.
**Feeding.** Nancy progressed from total parenteral nutrition (through the veins directly into the circulation near the heart) to gavage feeding (tube into the stomach) to alternate gavage and nipple and, finally, to nippling only.
**Temperature.** At first, Nancy had all the heat provided for her by the radiant warmer and then the incubator. She advanced to being able to maintain her temperature by intermittently leaving that heat source and eventually going to an open-air crib where she could maintain her temperature while normally swaddled.
**Weight.** Nancy progressed from losing some of her original birthweight to fluctuating between gains and losses to a continual, gradual gain of 5 grams per day. Once she started gaining 15 to 20 grams ($1/2$ to $2/3$ ounce), we knew she might consistently gain weight and we called her a "growing premie."

## YOUR PREMIE'S TUMULTUOUS NEW WORLD

The great advances in medicine and technology currently available in the NICU saved Nancy's life. But these breakthroughs are not without their costs.

Because a baby's senses are, for the most part, fully functioning at the time of birth (see Chapter 7, "Why Kangaroo

Care Works"), the environment of the NICU comes as quite a shock to her. It in no way resembles the world within the womb, being both overstimulating and overwhelming. Indeed, research has shown that although the procedures available in the modern, well-equipped NICU save babies' lives, they can be overwhelming in terms of a premie's ability to handle environmental stimulation.

Most of the stimulation in the NICU is nonreciprocal— that is, it occurs irrespective of a premie's needs at the time or his ability to handle it. The constant clamor, bright lights, and invasive procedures limit his opportunities for much-needed sleep and for socially reinforcing person-to-person, face-to-face contact. Chapter 13 discusses ways of shaping the NICU environment to make it more reciprocal to your infant's needs and abilities. Here let's consider the impact of normal NICU activity on the premie's senses and routines.

### SOUND

Within the womb, noise is filtered and muffled by muscle, fluid, and bone. Outside the womb, your premie's ears enjoy none of that protection. The noise level in the intensive care nursery is 10 to 22 decibels louder than that in the newborn nursery, ranging around 60 to 70 decibels at all times. (Normal speech is at 65 decibels.) At 70 decibels, sleep disturbances may begin to occur. If the sound level exceeds 84 decibels repeatedly over time, your child can experience a hearing loss from the sound's cumulative effects.

The din in the NICU has a wide variety of sources. The infant is assailed by the incessant beeping of other babies' monitor alarms, the excited voices of parents visiting neighboring incubators, the jangle of the phones, the grating of the addressograph, and the rattle of trash cans.

These sounds are quite loud. For example, the sound of shutting incubator portholes runs from 111 to 124 decibels. Setting a milk bottle down softly on top of an incubator measures from 84 to 100 decibels, closing the cabinet doors under the incubator from 104 to 119 decibels. The ambient noise level has been measured at between 50 to 68 decibels inside incubators even when the portholes are closed. When open, it's 60 to 68 decibels.

With this continuous racket, it should be no surprise that a number of babies suffer from hearing impairment when they leave the neonatal intensive care unit. To be certain that hearing loss is detected, most babies are given a hearing test before discharge. Most hearing loss is temporary.

Obviously, you want the environment around your baby to be as quiet as possible. In an attempt to find a solution to this problem, Dr. Lina Zahr of the University of California, Los Angeles, recently studied 46 premies wearing tiny earmuffs in the NICUs at UCLA Medical Center and Kaiser-Permanente Hospital in Los Angeles, California. Dr. Zahr learned that earmuffs do reduce the peak noise levels significantly (regularizing heart and breathing rates) but that some babies became uncomfortable wearing them over a long period of time. Dr. Zahr now recommends using earmuffs occasionally and implementing other noise-cutting strategies such as padding the incubator and keeping the incubator portholes closed during the noisiest parts of the shift, such as when care-givers go on medical rounds. (See Chapter 13, "Shaping the Intensive Care Nursery Experience.")

Clearly, the solution to the problem of excessive noise requires changes in the baby's environment, not just the use of ear protection. During Kangaroo Care babies fall so deeply asleep that they are able to shut out the noise.

## LIGHT

Bright lights are disturbing to young babies. You'll notice infants closing their eyes and turning their heads away when suddenly confronted with bright lights or sunshine.

But nurses need lighting to conduct their business—to check the babies' skin color, make sure all the equipment is functioning, take readings from the various monitors, get connectors together, write their notes, and so on. Radiant warmers emit illumination, which adds to the brightness if the lights are also on. Unfortunately, many older nurseries lack dimmer switches or baby-specific lamps (lamps turned on only when needed for a treatment).

Not only do bright lights disturb infants, but they can also permanently impair a child's visual abilities. As early as 1985, we learned that high levels of illumination in the NICU may actually damage premies' retinas and may possibly contribute to blindness.

More recently, many institutions have become quite conscious about turning down the lights. They have added baby-specific lamps and may even use eye patches to minimize light stimulation for a short period of time, as when the baby is going to be under a particularly bright light for a procedure. (Leaving eye patches on all the time is not a good idea, as it can produce visual deprivation in babies and creates the potential for amblyopia, or blurry vision.)

Ideally, you'll want your baby in a semidarkened environment similar to the womb.

*DAY-NIGHT CYCLING*

The activities in the NICU may continue unabated whether it's night or day. Yet, appropriate day-night cycling promotes the development of your premie's circadian rhythm. The circadian rhythm is the flux in hormones and metabolic rate to maximize the body's use of energy during periods of wakefulness or sleep. Development of a circadian rhythm will eventually help your infant adjust to your family's activities, and more important, it has repercussions for your infant's growth and development.

When the circadian rhythm is well-established, your infant's brain will modulate the output of growth hormone and other hormones that regulate body health and organ functioning. When sleep patterns are regularized, your infant will have regular surges in growth hormone and will be better able to tolerate changes in his environment. Unfortunately, the usual routines and hubbub in the NICU interfere with day-night cycling.

Kangaroo Care gives the infant more opportunities for sleep, which should promote circadian rhythm development.

## INVASIVE MEDICAL PROCEDURES

Medical touch refers to any touch related to therapy. Social touch, on the other hand, consists of soothing, calming, and affectionate behaviors. Most premies in the NICU, unfortunately, experience far more of the former than they do the latter. Medical care (heel sticks, intubations, daily weights and measures, chest physical therapy) is necessary but can be disruptive, interrupting the baby up to 130 times a day.

Researchers have found that with almost every form of medical touch, premies experience a series of physiological changes that indicate stress: infants' oxygen levels temporarily decrease, their heart rates decline, and the blood pressure in the brain increases. These changes stress babies even more!

Dr. Peter Gorski at the Northwestern University School of Medicine in Chicago has devoted much of his work to finding ways to protect the premie from the invasive environment— to allow these medical procedures to occur without compromising the baby's health. Dr. Gorski found that one key to helping babies deal with all the medical touch that's required is to consolidate it as much as possible and monitor the infants' responses to the treatments as they proceed, slowing as necessary.

Rather than disturbing the baby several times within the same hour—once for feeding, a second time for a blood test, a third time to suction the lungs—these procedures could be grouped together and performed at the same time or one after another. In addition, the nursing staff should look at the baby's heart and respiratory rates when the baby is calm and inactive and conduct the procedure only as long as the baby's basic data stay around this baseline.

In critical situations, it's impossible to follow these recommendations every time. Saving the baby's life is the health team's first job. Intensive care is, after all, intensive. Even though invasive procedures may have a short-term negative effect, the long-term outcome is to the baby's advantage. A premie will cry when her nurse inserts an IV, but without it, she won't get the antibiotic that will save her from an infection.

Ideally, you would want your infant to endure the necessary medical procedures with as little stress as possible. As you will see in the next several chapters, Kangaroo Care can help do just that.

## NURSERY SHUTDOWN

Researchers, nurses, and doctors have become aware of the problem of overstimulation of infants in the intensive care unit. Recently, they have attempted to find ways to alleviate the stress that such an overstimulating environment creates.

One of these techniques is called "nursery shutdown." It originated with Dr. Jerold Lucey, a neonatologist at the University of Vermont. Dr. Lucey is one of the first researchers credited with modifying the neonatal intensive care unit environment on behalf of newborns. His system shuts out all types of sensory overload for a specified period of time.

Here's how nursery shutdown works. For an hour or two during each shift, Dr. Lucey had the phone ringers disconnected, the beepers turned off, the alarms turned down, the radios silenced, the bright lights eliminated, the conversation kept to a minimum, and the ventilators padded to muffle the sound. During this period, the doors to the unit remained shut. All medically related touch, labwork, and treatments had to be finished before shutdown, so that the infants were left undisturbed. Nurses took vital signs from the equipment rather than by touching the infants.

The babies did beautifully under this system, and Dr. Lucey's idea has now spread around the country. The University of Colorado Medical Center has instituted a "nap time" throughout its intensive care unit. Other hospitals implement this system particularly at night. However the system is implemented, we have all learned from these studies that periods of shutdown are both feasible and advisable.

As you'll see, Kangaroo Care creates a natural form of nursery shutdown that's loving and restorative.

# 5

# Understanding Your Premie's Messages

Your baby is as aware of the NICU environment as you are! In fact, premies are quite adept at showing us what they think of the place and the treatment they're receiving, if we only know what to look for.

Only recently has the medical community realized that this is so. Until 1985, it was believed that premature babies felt no pain and therefore required no analgesics, even during surgery—a truly barbaric state of affairs! But once researchers recognized and began focusing on infants' pain, they reasoned that babies might exhibit signs of distress before actually starting to cry. And so they began a systematic evaluation of infants' behavioral and physical cues.

They were amazed to find that babies exhibit an entire repertoire of subtle but reliable signals indicating both distress and peacefulness. They also found that these behaviors change as the infant matures and is better able to decide which behavioral cues are most effective in eliciting a response.

As you visit your infant in the NICU, you can follow how he is progressing by observing his physiological and behavioral messages. I have found, however, that mothers and fathers approach their babies in intensive care quite differently.

# THE PARENT GENDER GAP IS REAL

Women seem to focus in on details. When a new mother calls to ask about her baby, she typically poses questions such as:

- How many ccs of milk did Rebecca take this morning?
- How many grams has she gained since yesterday?
- What percent of oxygen is she on today?
- How often does she get the antibiotic?
- Does she still need the blood transfusion? How much blood does she need?
- How many episodes of apnea (or bradycardia—slow heartbeat) has she had?
- How low did her heart rate go?
- Is she still on the theophylline? How much is she getting now?

Mothers demand precise numbers and chart the changes in their babies' health with minute and exact observations. They are also eager to learn what each piece of equipment does, what each number means, and how to tell if all the equipment is working properly. They learn the intensive care unit lingo quickly. They soon acquire what I like to think of as a Minor in Neonatology. They do a very fine job of keeping track of their infants' recovery.

Men, on the other hand, ask general questions like:

- How is Rebecca doing today?
- Is she breathing better?
- Is she eating more?
- Is she losing or gaining weight?
- Is she as sick as she was yesterday?

These global questions help them get the overall picture.

I find the differences in male and female behavior fascinating because parents complement each other's perspectives: One can see the forest for the trees; the other focuses on the roots, trunk, branches, and leaves. Together, they gain a whole picture of the child's progress.

But given a woman's response to her premie's medical care, it is little wonder that she quickly starts to differentiate each of her baby's behaviors. Indeed, soon she learns that her infant communicates her physiological and even mental state by sending various messages.

## HOW YOUR PREMIE "TALKS" TO YOU

You'll be amazed when you recognize your tiny premie's competence in communicating her likes and dislikes. Each infant is forced to endure all the forms of environmental input that deluge her. Your infant will communicate two types of messages to you, as she is confronted with environmental stimulation:

**Engagement:** "I'm handling everything OK, thank you."
**Time-out or distress:** "I'm a little overloaded. I can't handle what's going on around me. I need a break."

She communicates through changes both in her physiological state (monitored by her heart rate, respiratory rate, oxygen level, blood pressure, and skin color) and her behavioral signs. Let's consider each of these methods of infant communication.

## PHYSIOLOGICAL CHANGES

Watch your baby's monitors during a quiet, calm period. These readings will give you a baseline of her heart rate, respiratory rate, and oxygen levels. Changes in these rates are your premie's way of communicating how she is adapting to her environment.

*HEART RATE*

The younger the baby, the higher the heart rate; a range of 110 to 160 beats per minute is normal, depending on the infant's size. The baseline is established when the premie is lying quietly. Usually the rate can move up or down by 10 beats per minute with no ill effect. But if the heart rate suddenly changes 15 beats per minute (up or down) from the baseline, then we recognize that the infant is having trouble adapting.

Heart rates of 180 or more (severe tachycardia) indicate that your baby may have a fever, is stressed, or is crying and agitated. You will notice your baby's heart rate can go as high as 210 to 215 beats per minute with hard crying but it doesn't stay at that level. As soon as the crying stops, her heart rate should rapidly come back down to normal. In addition, if your infant is moving about in her bed, heart rates of 170 up to 190 may accompany her movement. Again, this decreases as soon as she becomes still.

Heart rates below 100 (severe *bradycardia*) may indicate fatigue, cold, very deep sleep, low oxygen levels, or difficulties maintaining heart rate. This is often due to brain immaturity. Bradycardia is dangerous because it impairs blood flow to the brain, thus depriving it of vital oxygen.

Your baby's brain is essential for life; it must be in optimal condition for her to grow and to overcome the problems associated with immaturity. The brain requires a consistent and steady supply of blood to get the oxygen it needs to perform properly. It responds poorly to increases or decreases in the frequency and pressure of blood flowing to it. The amount of blood that reaches the brain is governed, in part, by your premie's heartbeat, so stability of heart rate is of major concern.

You'll notice bradycardias often accompany feeding; until premies are closer to term and more mature, it's hard for them, especially when they're tired, to maintain their heart rate while sucking.

During Kangaroo Care, bradycardia has been markedly reduced and tachycardia is rarely seen.

*RESPIRATORY RATE*

The younger the baby, the higher the respiratory rate. The normal range for premature babies is 35 to 50 breaths per minute, but respiratory rates of 60 are quite common among babies under 1,500 grams (about 3 pounds). A sudden change of 10 breaths per minute (up or down) from the baseline indicates that your baby may have some trouble adapting.

Respiratory rates, like heart rates, will exceed the normal range when babies become active and agitated or when they cry. (Rates can be 60 breaths per minute or more during crying.) This is called *tachypnea*. During episodes of *bradypnea*, on the other hand, the respiratory rate drops below 30 breaths per minute. More shallow breathing patterns occur when your baby is in deep sleep or is calm and contented.

Low breathing rates, however, are quite different from not breathing at all. When your baby stops breathing, she is experiencing apnea. Apneas are important but only if they exceed 10 seconds in duration. Episodes under 10 seconds are common; usually your baby will spontaneously reverse and come out of it. If the apnea is 10 seconds or longer, however, medical staff intervene by touching the infant, holding her foot, putting a finger in her mouth, calling her name, and trying to arouse her to restart breathing. Extended episodes of apnea are dangerous and can lead to death.

Bradypnea and some apnea often occur as premies learn to coordinate their breathing with feeding. It's hard for them to do both at once! Interestingly, during Kangaroo Care even though infants go to the breast often, the incidence of apnea decreases dramatically.

*OXYGEN LEVELS*

Most parents quickly determine which piece of equipment indicates their baby's oxygen level. It's usually the pulse oximeter that gives the oxygen saturation level. (See Chapter 4, "Life in the Neonatal Intensive Care Unit.") This piece of equipment is extremely sensitive to movement. As you watch it, you'll notice that the numbers change as soon as your baby starts to move the part of her body to which it's attached. For baseline oxygen saturation level, you'll want to know what the percentage is over three consecutive minutes when your baby is quiet.

The normal oxygen saturation values for premies are 88 to 100 percent, although sometimes narrower ranges are desirable:

- If your baby is on a ventilator, we would want her oxygen saturation level to approximate a range near 90 to 94 percent.
- If your baby is receiving oxygen by hood, face mask, or cannula, we want the value to be 91 to 97 percent.
- If your baby is in an open-air crib and not on oxygen therapy, anywhere between 88 and 100 percent is acceptable, though percentages in the 90s are preferable.

If the oxygen saturation level drops below these values for one to two minutes, this is a sign of distress. During Kangaroo Care, oxygen saturation levels have been in the normal range, even in those babies who were having difficulty breathing, as manifested by grunting respirations (see Chapter 6).

*BLOOD PRESSURE*

Blood pressure determinations are usually recorded continuously when the umbilical catheter is in place. After its removal, blood pressure may be taken once every 5, 15, 30, or 60 minutes in sick infants, less often in healthier ones.

Blood pressure varies greatly according to a baby's medical condition and medications. It's best to ask the nurse about your baby's baseline blood pressure and what is considered the blood pressure "comfort range." If your baby's pressure exceeds that range, it's a sure sign that something is bothering her—she may have insufficient oxygen or she may be responding to a loud sound in the environment. Sudden changes of 10 millimeters of mercury in either the top or bottom number would indicate that your premie is responding unfavorably to the environment.

We haven't measured blood pressure during Kangaroo Care, because the inflating cuff can be irritating to premies. My best guess, however, is that blood pressure stays within normal range during Kangaroo Care, because the babies are so peaceful and at rest and often sleeping.

*SKIN COLOR*

Under the lights in the intensive care unit, your baby's skin usually won't appear pink. Rather, it will be more of a pale pink or, for African-American babies, light brown color. If your child has *jaundice,* her skin may appear yellow.

Skin color changes to red, dusky, blue, pale, or mottled indicate that your child is not adapting well to any and all forms of environmental stimulation.

During Kangaroo Care, your premie's skin should become pinker around the lips, in the palms, the face, and sometimes all the way down to the toes. This occurs because the warming of her skin up against your chest causes her blood vessels to dilate slightly. If you see your baby getting bluer, dusky, or pale during Kangaroo Care, it may be a sign that her oxygen level should be checked. Be sure that she has extensive skin-to-skin contact because as soon as she's off your chest even a little, her skin temperature will cool down and her skin can change color.

## BEHAVIORAL SIGNS OF DISTRESS

Your premie will also provide you with myriad behaviors that indicate how she is doing. But bear in mind that you are likely to see more distress than pleasure signs with a younger baby. Only as your premie nears 38 weeks postconceptual age will you start to see the signs of engagement described below that say, "I want to play. Keep me interested." And those you will welcome with all your heart!

The following are signs of distress to watch for while your baby is under a radiant warmer, in an incubator, or in an open-air crib:

1. *The white knuckle syndrome.* An infant normally holds her hands in a fist, but a premie under 32 weeks will probably hold her hands open when resting quietly. She doesn't have the muscle strength or tone to contract those muscles to form a fist. As your premie matures, you will notice that she gains the fisted posture of a full-term baby, flexing her fingers into her palm.

But although a fisted posture is common, a clenched fist is not. White knuckles are the result of a clenched fist. Even the youngest premie should not have white knuckles. I have found this indicates some sort of tension.

2. *Finger splay.* If you see your baby's fingers stretched out, recognize this as a sign of distress and tension. You want your infant to relax, cuddle up, and bend. The finger splay might begin suddenly but last a long time.

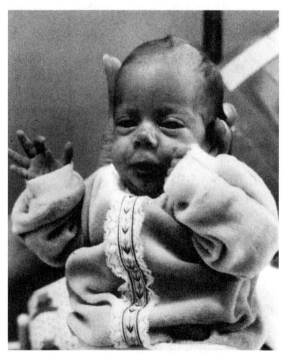

Finger splay

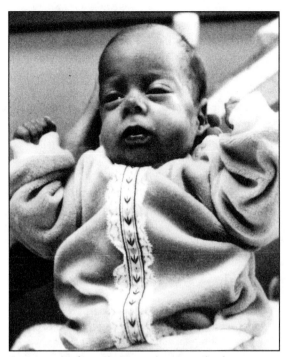
Sagging cheeks and chin and arching back

3. *Sagging cheeks and chin.* These are a sign of fatigue. They indicate that your baby doesn't have the energy to continue being exposed to whatever is happening to her. Her mouth may hang open and she may thrust out her tongue.

4. *Spitting up.* Spitting up may be sign of distress when it occurs, but some spitting up is inevitable because premies are poor feeders at first. If the regurgitation occurs during and right after a feeding, the probable cause is the immaturity of the valve between the esophagus and the stomach: it doesn't close tightly yet. (See the discussion of *gastroesophageal reflux* in Chapter 10, "Before, During, and After Kangaroo Care.") The nurse can help you distinguish stress-induced spitting up from that which is related to immaturity.

Whenever you see digesting food coming out of your baby's mouth, quickly turn her onto her stomach so she cannot swallow it back or choke on it. Lift her slightly from her bed so her mouth and nose aren't lying in it. Your premie may regurgitate even while you are breastfeeding her. If that happens, remove her from your breast and immediately turn her over, supporting her chest in one hand and patting her on the back with the other, as she lies facedown.

5. *Furrowed brow.* Look at your baby's brow as she is quiet and sleeping. Most likely it will be smooth. If she becomes worried, uneasy, or distressed, she will develop creases across the forehead, just as you would.

6. *Ear tuck.* I have found that when premies are relaxed, their ears stand away from their heads, but that under stressful situations, they tuck their ears back so that they're almost against the skull. I've observed this difference in premies from 32 weeks on. Prior to that, there's not enough cartilage and strength in the ear to have it stand away from the skull. Apparently we all lose this ability as we age.

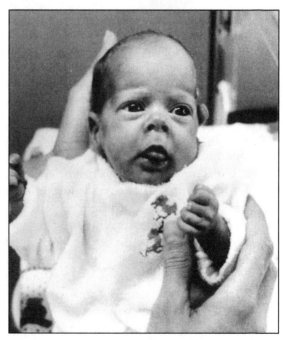

Furrowed brow and white knuckle syndrome. Notice left hand going up as a stop sign.

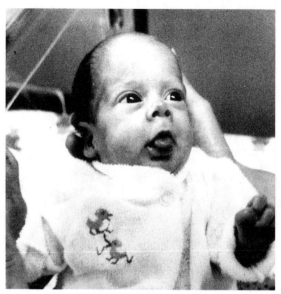

Ear tuck

7. *Stop sign.* A premie is quite competent at bending her arm at the elbow and putting her hand up, even if she's sleeping. The message is clear. Stop whatever is happening to me. I cannot take it anymore.

Don't confuse this movement with a startle, in which both arms move out to the periphery of your baby's body and then tremble as they come back toward the middle.

8. *Air sitting.* This is the lower extremity version of the stop sign. Your baby's legs go up as if she were doing a leg lift.

9. *Arching back.* Your baby starts to arch her back and pull away from the person who is holding her. She is trying to create physical distance and retreat from what she is encountering.

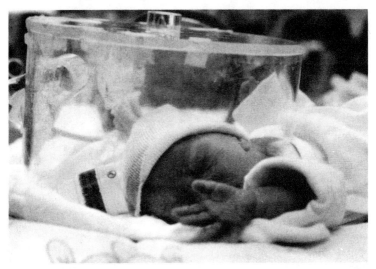

Stop sign

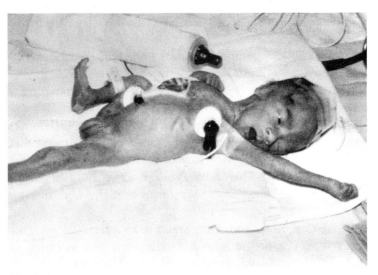

Air sitting

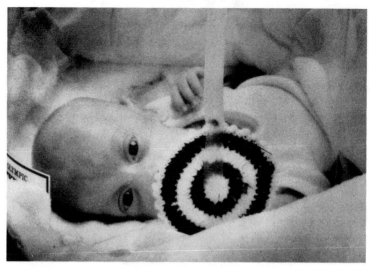

A premie gazing at his black-and-white toy.

10. *Hyperalertness.* When your premie is merely *awake*, her eyes are open. When she's *alert*, she is attentive; she concentrates on, thinks about, or mentally engages in whatever she is looking at. Usually when we see this alertness, we talk to our infant more, engage her, and show her interesting black-and-white designs. (These have been shown to be the only appropriate and visually appealing targets for premies and newborns under 6 months of age. See our book *How to Have a Smarter Baby* for instructions on how to use these targets.) We try to reinforce that attention span.

Sometimes babies become too tired to retreat. At this point, their attentiveness transforms into a stare, called a "hyperalert" state. If your premie becomes hyperalert, her eyes will be wide open. She'll be looking, but she'll seem a little fearful. You will be able to identify this in the pained expression on her face.

11. *Gaze aversion.* Your baby will turn her eyes away from whatever she was looking at or she'll shift her eyes from right to left. This is a sign of stress because your premie can't manage to handle what's happening in the environment; she can't keep her eyes focused on any one thing.

12. *Head turning.* If gaze aversion doesn't work and your

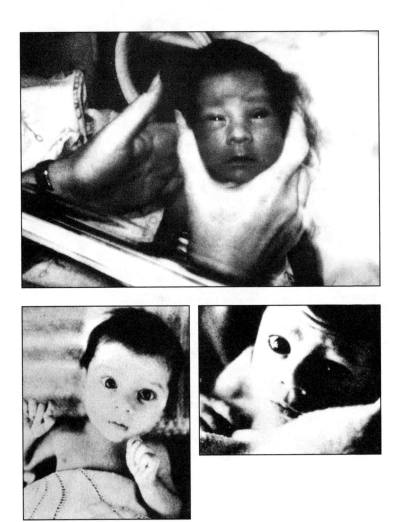

Here are examples of three levels of attentiveness: awake (top); alert (above left); hyperalert infant with furrowed brow (above right).

baby has enough tone in her neck muscles, she'll turn her whole head away. If she does so in a back-and-forth motion as if to say, "No, no!" we regard this response as a high level of activity and consequently distress.

13. *Yawning or hiccuping.* Both usually accompany fatigue or stress and are a sign that you must stop whatever activity is going on. We tend to ignore yawns, but they mean please back off.

14. *Tactile reinforcement.* This behavior involves your baby touching herself in order to withdraw from the environment. The touch message is very strong and is believed to compete with outside stimuli for perception in the brain. In this way it distracts your child from an unwanted activity.

Your infant may touch herself in many ways. She will put her thumb on her index finger. If she needs stronger self-consoling, she will touch one hand to the other. Many babies need to do this to get themselves to sleep and maintain sleep. It's something they can do for themselves. If when you're interacting with your premie, you see this tactile reinforcement, stop what you're doing. (But let her continue with her tactile reinforcement to maintain her sleep.)

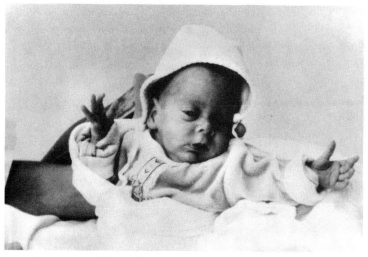

An infant turning his head and averting his gaze.

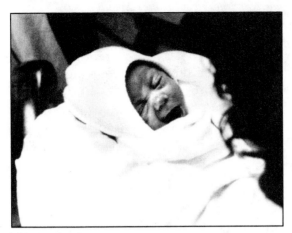

This is what happens . . .

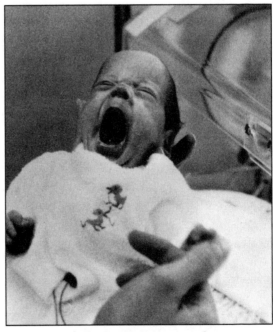

. . . when a person doesn't honor an infant's yawns.

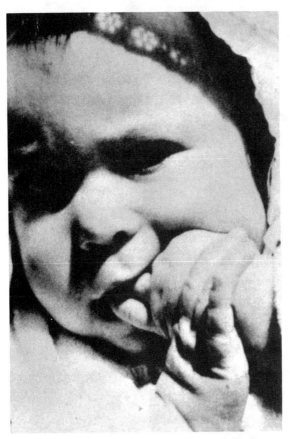

Tactile reinforcement. Infant touching one hand to
the other.

In the most extreme cases, your infant will bring both
hands up to her mouth to shut out the environment. If she
does that, she may begin sucking on her fingers, a positive and
powerful form of self-consoling, which we encourage. (See
Chapter 11, "Breastfeeding During Kangaroo Care," for an
explanation of the benefits of nonnutritive sucking.)

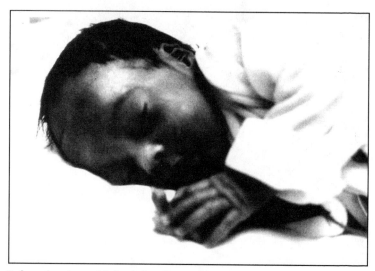

Infant sleeping with both hands touching.

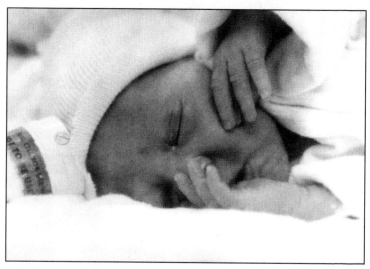

Infant putting his hands up to his mouth while asleep in an effort to console himself.

## WHAT TO DO IF YOU RECOGNIZE SIGNS OF DISTRESS

The signs of distress all indicate that your premie is experiencing tension, discomfort, or malaise. We have not seen these behaviors in premies during Kangaroo Care, but they do occur when babies are under radiant warmers and in incubators or open-air cribs or being transferred into and out of Kangaroo Care.

Inez Verzemnieks, a doctoral student at UCLA's School of Nursing, developed a handy system to teach parents how to react appropriately when babies exhibit distress cues. She calls her system SORTE. Just follow the simple SORTE steps when you recognize your baby's distress cues in the intensive care unit.

**S: Stop** whatever is happening to her at that moment. (She's being stroked or turned, people are talking around her, alarms are going off, and so on.)

**O: Offer** a hand or a voice. Place one hand over the top of her head or on her abdomen or thigh without movement. (This action contains the baby.) Try to soothe your infant with your calm, caressing voice. Quietly maintain this action for about one minute.

**R: Readjust** your infant's position. Flex her legs at the knees and tuck her feet in under her and/or hold her arms in to cover her chest.

**T: Try** again whatever activity took place when your baby became distressed.

**E: End** whatever you were doing if baby becomes distressed after a second or third attempt.

The key here is to respect your infant's need for pauses in her activity and an acceptable level of stimulation. Remember, though, because she's a premie, it takes time for her brain to organize all the messages required to shape behavior. She may need 30 seconds to 2 minutes to organize her behavior to stop crying and get her normal breathing rate back. This is called *latency to respond,* since she must take time to process the input and change her behavior.

## BEHAVIORAL SIGNS OF HAPPINESS

Your baby will also give you many signs that she's happy. In general these are the opposite of the negative signs and include:

- A relaxed brow
- Uplifted cheeks and chin
- Gently flexed hand
- A flexed posture
- A smile

In Kangaroo Care you will see smiles, relaxed inactivity, and a look of utter contentment. With multiple sessions of Kangaroo Care, your baby will probably awaken and turn her head to search for your face. She may look from 4 to 10 seconds and then close her eyes, pause to recuperate her ability to attend, and look at you again.

# 6

# Why You Should Use Kangaroo Care

We know that Kangaroo Care has an extraordinary effect on premature babies. But through what mechanism does Kangaroo Care have this extraordinary effect? Does Kangaroo Care work primarily by affecting a particular organ system— for example, the nervous system, the heart and lungs, the urinary tract, or the gastrointestinal tract? Is the mechanism primarily behavioral? Or, does Kangaroo Care work through a psychophysiological cascade of effects that simply evade definition?

Research on Kangaroo Care conducted around the world quickly revealed that it influences many organ systems and behaviors at once. Kangaroo Care improves the premie's:

- Body temperature
- Heart rate
- Breathing patterns and oxygen saturation
- Weight and growth
- Behavioral state (sleep and alertness)
- Emotional state
- Breastfeeding patterns (see Chapter 11)
- Bonding (see Chapter 2)

Now that you know Kangaroo Care is a valuable therapy, let's look at its benefits in greater detail.

## BODY TEMPERATURE

Staying warm is of the utmost importance to your baby. Warmth helps your premie sleep. It also enables him to use his calories more efficiently. Rather than having to generate his own heat, he can devote his limited energy resources to the vital tasks of repair and maturation of his tissues. Body temperature is regulated by the *thermoregulatory system:* the hypothalamus, blood vessels, skin, and sweat glands.

Just as Drs. Rey and Martínez theorized, a mother's skin temperature helps her baby stay warm during Kangaroo Care. Research has established incontrovertibly that when a mother holds her baby and there are *proper controls over what covers the infant's back, the airflow, and environmental temperature,* that baby will stay warm.

Nevertheless, many physicians still ask, "Won't a baby who is completely nude become cold? How can a mother be as warm as an incubator or a radiant warmer?" In truth, premies aren't nude during Kangaroo Care; they stay warm when properly covered with a diaper and blanket. In Chapter 10, "Before, During, and After Kangaroo Care," you will find a discussion of appropriate attire for your infant during Kangaroo Care.

Premies who are quite sick and consequently have been placed under radiant warmers have not yet been rigorously studied in Kangaroo Care. On the other hand, many investigations have been carried out with comparably low birthweight but healthier babies who are in incubators. These babies all stayed warm during Kangaroo Care.

Older, bigger babies who have subcutaneous fat layers and a good supply of brown fat tissue (this develops in the last month of gestation), which help them to generate their own heat, are able to maintain the proper temperature during Kangaroo Care. Interestingly, even the smaller babies discussed above who do not have that all-important fat tissue have also been able to stay toasty. They, too, warm up to a *neutral thermal zone* (the temperature range at which a baby has minimal oxygen needs).

Usually the warming follows a specific pattern: The baby's temperature rises quickly for the first 10 minutes and then stabilizes within the neutral thermal zone for the remainder of the kangarooing session. In tropical climates, in rare instances, babies continue the warming process as the session continues. An excessive body temperature will burn calories, use up oxygen, speed up metabolic processes, and create breathing problems. For this reason, in these climates we recommend checking the infant's temperature more frequently. In Chapter 10, I will explain how to cool your baby, but this information is rarely needed.

In general, as Kangaroo Care continues within a session, incubator babies who have more immature thermoregulatory systems gradually become warmer. In a three-hour session of Kangaroo Care, the incubator babies who have been studied have not exceeded the normal temperature range (37.5° centigrade, 99.5° Fahrenheit skin temperature). This is encouraging because it suggests that even with a more immature thermoregulatory system, Kangaroo Care does not overheat the baby.

## HEART RATE

Taking advantage of the continuous monitoring in the premature nursery, in our research we found that during Kangaroo Care heart rate remained relatively stable around a baseline. It consistently hovered around 140 to 160 plus or minus 5 beats. As an infant sleeps in Kangaroo Care, her heart rate can become quite regular.

Cardiac stability means that the blood vessels become accustomed to a regular rate of blood flow and that all of the tissues are being fed at a regular, stable rate. With less variability of heart rate, the brain also receives a steady supply of life-sustaining oxygen.

When your baby awakens or cries, her heart rate can soar above 160 and even as high as 215 if she is crying hard. As you can imagine, a fluctuating heart rate is difficult for the baby to maintain. We like to keep her heart rate regular, and that's what you'll achieve in Kangaroo Care.

You can anticipate that your premie's heart rate will increase by 5 to 10 beats per minute during Kangaroo Care. This is normal and expectable: As her body warms, her heart rate increases. It's also significant that your baby may not experience a drop in heart rate (bradycardia). Even babies still in incubators have not experienced bradycardia during Kangaroo Care.

# RESPIRATORY RATE

One of the primary focuses of the medical team in the neonatal intensive care unit is to establish a baby's regular breathing. There are many noninvasive ways to measure your premie's respiratory function. Care-givers can look at the respiratory rate and the entire breathing pattern (the depth of breathing: shallow versus deep) as well as at episodes of apnea (periods in which the premie "forgets" to breathe) and rapid, deep breaths. Care-givers can also measure how much oxygen the blood actually contains. Let's look more closely at these ways of measuring respiratory function.

## BREATHING PATTERNS

Before Kangaroo Care your baby's breathing rate might have ranged from 15 breaths per minute up to 60 breaths per minute, depending on her level of activity and arousal. Activity and increasing awakeness cause your infant to consume more oxygen. She must meet her increasing oxygen needs by breathing more frequently.

During Kangaroo Care, on the other hand, your baby is likely to have a normal respiratory rate of 35 to 50 breaths per minute. Her breathing pattern most likely will improve over what it was when she was lying in the crib or incubator.

In our research, and that of others, it has been found that:

- The depth of each breath becomes more even.
- Apnea decreases fourfold or is entirely absent.

- The length of any apnea episode diminishes.
- *Periodic breathing* (a situation in which apnea alternates with huge catch-up breaths, followed by other episodes of apnea) decreases significantly.

It is clear that Kangaroo Care helps to stabilize a premie's breathing.

### OXYGEN IN THE BLOOD

It's fine to know that all of these breathing patterns are improving, but the real test of Kangaroo Care comes in determining how much oxygen actually makes its way into the baby's blood. There are two easy ways to measure this. The first is called *transcutaneous* (through the skin) *pressure of oxygen.* You may hear this referred to in the neonatal intensive care unit as *TCPO$_2$.* In this procedure, care-givers measure the pressure of oxygen traveling in the blood cells right under the skin. A sensor is placed on the infant's skin with a gel. This warms the skin and dilates the blood vessels under it so that the pressure of oxygen in the blood can be measured as it passes under the sensor.

All studies have shown that the pressure of oxygen in the blood cells increases during Kangaroo Care even when the session is as short as ten minutes!

The second method is to discover the oxygen saturation level of the blood cells. (See Chapter 4, "Life in the Neonatal Intensive Care Unit.") Oxygen saturation rarely diminishes during Kangaroo Care (and only when overheating begins) and has even seen slight improvement. In fact, even with incubator babies, oxygen levels below normal range have rarely been seen.

If your baby is on a carbon dioxide monitor, during Kangaroo Care you will probably see a drop in the value of carbon dioxide and a corresponding rise in that of oxygen. This, too, is a positive sign.

From research done to date, it is clear that oxygenation of the blood throughout the body, all the way out to the fingertips and toes, is not threatened during Kangaroo Care.

## RESPIRATORY DISTRESS

Kangaroo Care appears to helps reduce respiratory distress. In 1992, Dr. Gene Cranston Anderson and I went to the Hospital Universitario del Valle, Cali, Colombia, to study the use of Kangaroo Care immediately after birth. Kangaroo Care had been so salutary for older babies, it seemed logical to test its benefits when begun sooner.

There can be a problem beginning Kangaroo Care so early, however. Some premies automatically develop breathing problems shortly after birth. Their breaths become labored and audible. These early signs of respiratory distress are called *grunting respirations*. Babies emit these sounds as they instinctively try to prevent their lungs from collapsing by retaining some air within the passageway. When a premie develops grunting respirations, he is usually taken to the NICU and respirator tubes are put down his throat. His lungs are inflated artificially, using CPAP. (See Chapter 4, "Life in the Neonatal Intensive Care Unit.")

Dr. Anderson believed that Kangaroo Care could alleviate respiratory distress in premies. During her doctoral work on newborn sheep at the University of Wisconsin, she had found that when a lamb stays with his mother and the ewe is allowed to hold him against her body and lick him, he unexpectedly recovers from breathing difficulties. "Why not let the baby stay with his mother and see if her warmth and contact have the same effect?" she suggested.

Dr. Anderson appealed to Dr. Humberto Rey (no relation to Dr. Edgar Rey), the Chairman of the Department of Pediatrics at the hospital, to permit us to try Kangaroo Care with a premie who developed grunting respirations. Although he was reluctant at first, he allowed Dr. Anderson to demonstrate the technique for him and his pediatric staff. When Dr. Rey and his staff saw how the infant warmed, how his oxygen saturation improved, and how peaceful and at rest he was, they became eager to have us continue.

We soon encountered a premie who experienced respira-

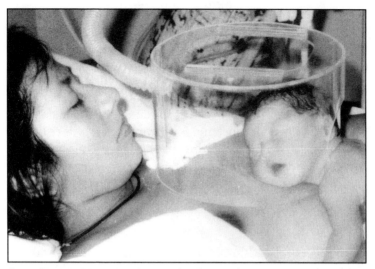

A newborn in Kangaroo Care under an oxygen tent.

tory distress and tried Dr. Anderson's approach again. We placed an oxygen hood over this baby as he lay on his mother's chest in Kangaroo Care. Initially the grunting respirations became louder, but soon they subsided. By six hours after birth, all signs of respiratory distress had disappeared. As expected and hoped for, the infant did beautifully.

We believed that the respiratory distress was resolved through the combined action of the warm, humidified oxygen together with the mother's warmth (which helped the baby to conserve his oxygen), the respiratory regulation that develops from contact with the mother, and the contentment, relaxation, and sleep that accompany Kangaroo Care.

We subsequently studied 14 newborns with respiratory distress; these newborns were all 34 to 36 weeks postconception. We found that when warm humidified oxygen was given by hood as the baby reclined in Kangaroo Care on the mother's chest, the respiratory distress ended within eight hours. All 14 infants in our study were sent to the postpartum unit—they never needed the NICU—and were discharged home within 48 hours.

## WEIGHT AND GROWTH

Overall growth—not just weight gain—may improve during Kangaroo Care. In part, that's because the premie is resting in a contained position; snuggling into your breast, he experiences fewer *random startles*. He becomes so content being held in this manner that he will quiet and for the most part will cease any restless fidgeting. He is burning fewer calories while he's quiet. Most likely, he'll go to sleep. During sleep, oxygen and calorie consumption are at their lowest levels. Your baby will be saving these precious calories for weight gain.

Over and over again researchers have documented that during Kangaroo Care, babies go to the breast and suckle. With successful suckling, they should increase their intake of calories and consequently grow and gain weight. Older premies enjoying Kangaroo Care have gained more than 15 to 20 grams (1/2 to 2/3 ounce) per day.

Continuous, repetitive daily weight gains of even 10 to 15 grams are good news. Commonly babies lose weight in the NICU before they become medically stable. With Kangaroo Care, we anticipate that if they're losing weight, they'll begin to gain weight, and that if they're already gaining weight, the weight gain will increase.

## BEHAVIORAL STATES

Like normal full-term infants, your premie experiences twelve levels of arousal (called "behavioral states"). These twelve levels are regular quiet sleep, irregular quiet sleep, active sleep, very active sleep, drowsiness, alert inactivity, quiet awake, awake active, awake very active, fussy, cry, and hard cry. Kangaroo Care has a positive effect on the appearance of desirable states (such as quiet, regular sleep) and on the reduction of undesirable states (such as awake very active) in premies in the intensive care unit.

### SLEEP

While he was still in utero, your infant slept from 20 to 22 hours a day. He enjoyed a deep sleep. But now in the neonatal intensive care nursery, it is common for him to grab only 2 hours of deep, quiet regular sleep—at the most—per day, commonly taken in 10- to 20-second bursts. During this type of sleep, his breathing is regular, his heart rate varies little, and his body is quiet, conserving energy.

The rest of your infant's time in the nursery is spent awake or in active sleep. During active sleep, though his eyes are closed, he is still moving about, wasting energy in purposeless activity. He is constantly awakened by environmental events such as medical procedures, bright lights, and loud noises. Anyone who watches a baby in an incubator will recognize that he gets very little deep, restorative sleep.

Before you begin Kangaroo Care, observe your baby. Most likely, you'll notice periods in which he's moving his fingers and toes, straightening his legs, twitching his face, making sucking motions, and fluttering his eyelashes, all while his eyes are closed. He may awaken quickly, cry, and try to get back to sleep. He is active and sleeping irregularly.

If you watch closely, you'll also note very short periods in which all of these activities have stopped. This is quiet, regular sleep. This kind of deep sleep is quite important, for it is at these moments that the brain is active in its own maturation process. During such slumber, your infant will be oblivious to environmental events such as bright lights and ringing telephones. Deep sleep reduces the baby's stress and is regenerating and refreshing. In addition, when your infant is in this state, his regular breathing will promote good blood oxygenation.

Research with premies in the intensive care unit has shown that babies spend most of their time in active sleep. But rather than accepting this as a norm, I believe we can help infants have deep, restorative sleep by using Kangaroo Care.

Babies sleep more frequently and for longer periods during Kangaroo Care. They go to sleep twice as often and have more than two and a half times the quiet, regular sleep when they're being held than when they're placed in their incubators or cribs. While in Kangaroo Care, your baby may go down into deep sleep and may stay there for 13 to 26 consecutive minutes. It's really wonderful rest.

It usually takes a baby five minutes to settle into this profound sleep. You can tell that he has reached this state because his hands and face will relax and his body will become heavier as you support it. Rather than twitching about as he had in the incubator, he may get himself into a position that he enjoys and may stay there comfortably and calmly.

Since sleep is one of the most significant remedies you can provide your infant, it's important to help him experience long, deep sleep episodes. Only if he gets enough sleep will he be able to be alert when it's important for him to be so (at

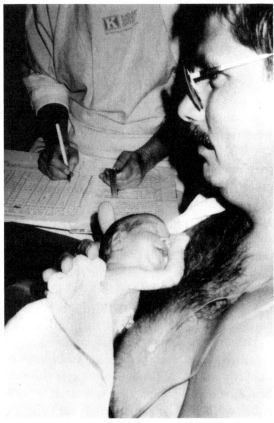

A Kangaroo Care baby rewards her father with a Mona Lisa smile.

around 38 weeks postconception) in order to interact with you as he gets ready to go home.

*ALERTNESS*

Alert inactivity refers to periods when your baby's eyes are open, he's attentive to something, and he's not moving his body purposelessly. Premies can see objects 10 to 13 inches from their faces. If they are more than 32 weeks postconception, they can see the object relatively clearly and can sustain their gaze for a few seconds. In general, premies will try to gaze on an object if it has light and dark contrast. Attentiveness is an advanced skill that usually can't be sustained longer than 4 to 10 seconds until the baby is at least 40 weeks postconception.

Following frequent Kangaroo Care, the duration of alertness increases markedly. When your infant has had several Kangaroo Care experiences, he will eventually, on awakening, start searching out your face. He may even crane his neck to locate your voice or to initiate eye-to-eye contact. (But you should not expect this reaction on your first few Kangaroo Care visits. You do want your baby to get his deep sleep.)

This response is rewarding for you and your baby alike and is necessary to foster good bonding, especially with the premature infant from whom you may have been separated a great deal.

*ACTIVITY*

In prematures, activity refers to purposeless movements or restless fidgeting. The infant's central nervous system is still too immature to filter out or dampen changes in her environment that might upset her. Instead, she experiences an all-or-nothing response unless she is in very deep sleep.

For example, if you should accidentally knock into your baby's incubator, you will immediately notice the following:

- Her heart rate increases.
- Her breathing speeds up.
- Her skin changes from pink to mottled to blue.

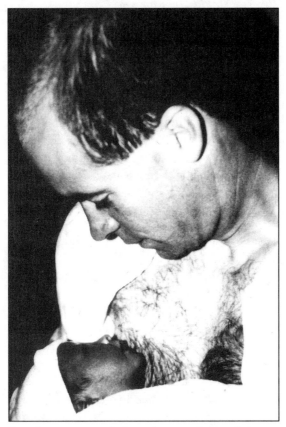

Premies can crane their necks to seek out their parents' faces during Kangaroo Care.

- She twitches all of her extremities: her legs, arms, hands, fingers.
- Her chest heaves.
- Her head turns.
- She grimaces.
- Her cheeks lift.

These responses eat up valuable oxygen and calories and can continue unabated for up to two minutes. As your baby becomes accustomed to the disturbance, the number of body changes will decrease.

When your premie is in Kangaroo Care, if you tap her on the shoulder or if someone makes a noise nearby, you will notice an absence of these dramatic reactions. A facial twitch, a finger extension, or a slight movement of a leg may be her only response, and even this will be short-lived. Your baby will continue to rest calmly without awakening. In Colombia, we noticed that even when we were taking blood from babies held in Kangaroo Care, not all infants would cry. Some tolerated this stressful procedure much better when their mothers held them.

During one of our research studies, we watched and measured the amount of time premies spent in purposeless, agitated movement during a period of 9 to 12 hours (including approximately 3 hours before Kangaroo Care, 3 hours during the session, and 3 hours after it). Predictably, we discovered that the infants spent significantly fewer minutes in an agitated state while in Kangaroo Care than while in their incubators or cribs or than other babies who did not receive Kangaroo Care.

## CRYING

The most awake behavioral state is called "hard crying." During this state, your baby's face gets red. His wailing is lusty and is accompanied by an increase in heart and respiratory rates. He may flail his arms and legs and grimace. A lot goes on during hard crying.

In the intensive care nursery, care-givers try to keep crying at a minimum. Despite their best attempts, crying in open-air cribs or incubators can go on for two to three minutes until exhaustion sets in or someone comes over to tend to the baby. But in Kangaroo Care, the number of crying episodes is significantly reduced and many babies don't cry at all. If they do cry, they usually recover within 60 seconds.

What crying we have seen hasn't been in response to distress about being placed in the kangaroo position. It has occurred prior to a feeding, as a sign that the baby is getting hungry. Fortunately, in Kangaroo Care, you can respond to that wail as soon as it appears. Your baby won't have to wait for the nurse to finish with another infant before tending to his needs. Be prepared, though: crying may occur when your baby is removed from Kangaroo Care, because he doesn't want to be taken from his safe, comfortable nest.

Interestingly, research findings indicate that premature babies who had experienced Kangaroo Care in the nursery cried significantly less at the age of 6 months than non–Kangaroo Care babies: 25 minutes per day rather than 38.

Very little if any crying occurs during Kangaroo Care because babies are happy to snuggle on their parents' chests and because they sleep so much. Rather than being agitated, these babies are relaxed and contented. This is critical, because crying is detrimental to premies in many ways:

- It increases pressure in the brain and can cause brain hemorrhages (strokes) that will retard an infant's development.
- It shunts blood through special heart valves that were needed during the fetal period. This prevents the blood from becoming oxygenated by diverting it from the lungs.
- It prevents the openings in the heart from closing quickly as they should so that the baby can grow.
- It causes oxygen levels in the blood to drop.
- It increases stress in babies.
- It is an immunosuppressant. That is, it puts an increased demand on the bone marrow to produce white blood cells at a rate which it cannot achieve.
- It contributes to air in the stomach, which can cause colic, increased irritability, and in severe cases, gastric rupture.

If your baby cries during Kangaroo Care, he is communicating a need rather than responding to distress.

## EMOTIONAL STATES

One of the most powerful observations you'll make during Kangaroo Care is how relaxed, contented, and calm your infant looks. I've watched many premies smile as they fall asleep, spontaneously awaken, smile again, and drift off back into deep slumber. And I've listened to mothers talk about how happy their babies seem to be while being held.

"Smile?" you may be thinking. "Premies don't smile. Even newborns can't smile yet. It must be gas!"

I'd like to respond to that old chestnut. Smiles during infancy are usually accompanied by a social purpose. A baby may smile to keep his parents playing with him or in response to some social interaction. While it is true that social smiling (in response to your talking and cooing to your infant) usually doesn't occur until a baby is 46 weeks postconception, during Kangaroo Care infants seem to smile quite deliberately. They can sustain the expression for up to a minute.

In contrast, reflex or gas-induced smiles are transient, fading after several seconds. Our research team has seen smiling in so many babies who have not had gas (or bowel movements, for that matter) that I am convinced these smiles are unrelated to gastrointestinal functioning. The fact that the smiling premie's heart and respiratory rates remain so stable also makes it highly unlikely that these smiles could be gas induced.

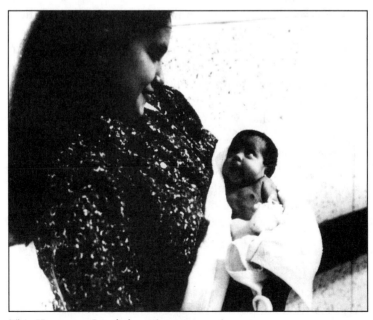

This Kangaroo Care baby is happy to go home!

Kangaroo Care smiles differ from social smiles. In general, smiling takes effort—a person must contract his facial muscles to communicate pleasure. By contrast, the Kangaroo Care smile seems effortless, and its purpose is not social. It usually occurs when the baby's eyes are closed. I believe it's a reflection of the infant's unconscious neurobehavioral enjoyment and an overall expression of his pleasure. It is motivated by his safe, warm, comfortable position, as if his central nervous system were saying, "This is great."

Happiness is a difficult variable to measure scientifically! I've watched these babies, and intuitively, I know they are happy. Nevertheless, I've often wondered how to quantify their pleasure.

Rather than using a relatively complex electroencephalogram (EEG) to measure brain wave patterns or computing the uplifted movement of premie's cheeks by calculating the action potential of muscle fibers, I decided to simply observe and count the number of smiles of whatever intensity during Kangaroo Care.

Today we are counting premie smiles at Kadlec Medical Center in Richland, Washington, with incubator babies getting Kangaroo Care and at the Hospital Maternidad in San Salvador, El Salvador, with open-air crib babies who receive Kangaroo Care beginning within a half hour of birth.

I am happy to report that we have observed smiling in Kangaroo Care that we have not seen when babies are in incubators or cribs. Of course, some babies don't smile at all but others have smiled three or four times during a one- or two-hour Kangaroo Care session. It's a really special feeling to know that you've been able to make a premature infant smile in the difficult situation of the neonatal intensive care unit.

## EARLY DISCHARGE FROM THE HOSPITAL

Because of all of these physiological and emotional benefits, it is not surprising that Kangaroo Care babies are being transferred from incubator to open-air cribs sooner and ultimately spend less time in the hospital. This not only saves money but, more important, also spares both parents and child emotional and physical wear and tear.

In an ongoing study, we compared two sets of incubator babies whose breathing tubes had been removed: those who had received five consecutive days of Kangaroo Care and those only cared for in incubators. Ironically, comparisons became difficult because the Kangaroo Care babies were being transferred to open-air cribs only three days after the mother-baby sessions began. None of these babies returned to incubators, and all were able to tolerate the transition without problems.

We also observed early discharge with babies in Cali, Colombia, who started Kangaroo Care in the delivery room. These infants were 34 to 37 weeks gestation at birth. Their APGARs at 5 minutes after birth were 6 or more (completely healthy infants have APGARs of 9 or 10), which indicated that they needed neither oxygen tubes in their throats nor placement in incubators. (See Chapter 8, "Is Your Baby Eligible for Kangaroo Care?")

We laid these babies on the mothers' chests in the delivery room as early as 12 minutes after birth and asked the women to hold them in Kangaroo Care for 6 hours. All of the babies tolerated the procedure well, and mothers and infants were transferred to a normal postpartum ward at the end of the six-hour period. All mothers and infants were discharged without complications after 24 to 48 hours.

Ms. Brigitte Syfrett, collaborating with Dr. Anderson, used the same procedure in the United States at Shands Hospital at the University of Florida and allowed mothers to continue Kangaroo Care for 2–3 days. Their preliminary finding is that Kangaroo Care babies go home at 3.7 days while similar babies sent to the intensive care unit go home at 10 days of life.

All in all, Kangaroo Care is a symphony of positive events. The baby is engulfed in his mother's or father's arms. He gains a sense of contentment. That relaxation and security accompanied by increasing warmth put him to sleep. The sleep cuts down on his agitation and purposeless activity, allowing him to utilize his calories for growth. It also places less demand on the heart and the breathing, so that these become more regular and unlabored. That leads to better oxygenation of the blood, which helps the brain mature to fight infections, establish a good sleeping pattern, and control the heart and breathing.

As the mother sees how her baby sleeps and relaxes in her presence, she becomes more content and less stressed over the birth. Consequently, she is more likely to have a milk letdown during Kangaroo Care. The scent of the milk attracts the baby, who is so close and who initiates a successful feeding experience. What a joy for all involved!

# 7

# Why Kangaroo Care Works

Although we now know that Kangaroo Care works, we are still speculating as to the reasons *why*. After untold hours of research and observation, I have come to the conclusion that this loving "treatment" is so effective because it contains some of the elements to which your baby grew accustomed while in the womb, providing an intimate form of protection so that healing rest and growth occurs. In this chapter, I'll explore with you why I believe this to be true.

## THE WORLD WITHIN THE WOMB

Most of us have the illusion that the world within the womb is a quiet, dark place where the fetus floats in serene tranquillity. Actually, nothing could be further from the truth. In our book *How to Have a Smarter Baby*, Susan Golant and I explain that the womb is a dynamic environment in which the fetus's developing senses receive all kinds of gentle stimulation.

For example, the nerve supply to the fetal ear is completed by the twenty-eighth week of gestation. The ear canal is open and the fetal brain responds to sounds by the thirty-fifth week. Since amniotic fluid conducts sound, your baby had been listening to your digestive gurglings, swallowing, heartbeat, and blood pulsations from that point on. These came through to his ear at a loud 72 to 84 decibels. (We talk to each other face-to-face at 65 decibels.) Mother's speech is distinguishable in utero despite the muffling caused by the tissues and organs separating the vocal cords from the fetus's ears.

The optic nerve, which transmits light from the eye to the brain, is formed by the eighth week of gestation. The fetal brain first responds to light at 27 weeks. Research has shown that the fetus's heart rate increases (indicating that he responds) when bright lights are shone on the mother's abdomen.

Your fetus will also have developed a sense of movement. The vestibule of the ear, the organ that senses movement, is formed by the seventeenth week of gestation, and the nerve responsible for transmitting the sense of movement matures by the twenty-fourth week. While the fetus is in utero, he will have experienced your natural movements such as standing, walking, bending, and rotating. As you move about, the amniotic sac rocks and rolls with you. Your breaths (normally 12 to 16 per minute) cause gentle waves within the sac.

During the first half of pregnancy, your fetus is floating free within the amniotic sac. He is able to bend his body, arms, and legs in gravity-defying feats, and he's been sucking his thumb as early as 7 weeks gestation. As gestation progresses, he sinks to the bottom of the womb and begins to fill the space. The uterine environment becomes increasingly snug until the fetus is no longer able to move about freely. Rather, arms and legs flexed in the "fetal position" as a result of his improved muscle tone, he is embraced within the bounds of a warm, safe, containing environment.

## A DÉJÀ VU OF THE WOMB

Kangaroo Care temporarily removes your premie from the stressful environment within the NICU described in Chapter 4 and in some ways re-creates for him the soothing comforts he enjoyed within the womb.

### MOTHER'S HEARTBEAT SOUNDS

When he's lying on your chest, your premie probably hears the same regular beat he heard through the womb. Heartbeat sounds are calming to newborns. We know that when we play tape recordings of these sounds to them, they stop crying and fall asleep. They may even turn their heads to better hear the sound. In fact, nurses may play tape recordings of heartbeat sounds in the Neonatal Intensive Care Unit to reduce babies' stress and help them sleep. These recordings are usually successful soporifics.

### SOUND OF MOTHER'S VOICE

The mother's familiar voice, which the fetus heard through the uterine wall, is comforting after birth. In scientific experiments, it was found that a newborn will alter his sucking patterns to turn on a tape recording of his mother's voice repeating the phrases she had used while he was in womb and will choose a tape of his mother's voice over a strange woman's voice.

Although to your fetus your voice was garbled, he could perceive its frequency, pitch, and tone. As your baby rests on your chest in Kangaroo Care, your voice may come through with some distortion, but its transmission remains the same even though it's traveling through bone and skin rather than muscle and fluid.

### ROCKING

Your premie enjoys gentle, rhythmic rocking as he rests on your chest. In the womb, your baby felt gentle undulations in the amniotic fluid as you breathed. Now as he rests on your chest he rocks at the same rate and with the same subtlety.

### SUCKING

From the seventh week of gestation, your fetus began to suck her fingers or any other body part she could get near her mouth. The sucking was necessary for her jaw and chin development so she would be ready to nurse at birth. Sucking is a strong need, and I believe it provides a sense of security.

As she lies in the incubator, it is very difficult for your premie to get her hands near her mouth. She doesn't have the muscle tone or strength to do so. It's almost equally impossible to get a pacifier to stay in her mouth. She may move her head about and suck with different strengths. A big suck pulls the pacifier in whereas a weak one pushes it out. She doesn't have a nipple readily available.

In Kangaroo Care, however, it's a short distance to the nipple. Your premie can suck on demand and on desire to soothe, comfort, and feed herself. (See Chapter 11, "Breast-feeding During Kangaroo Care.")

## CONTAINMENT

Containment was a predominant feature of the uterine environment, especially after 20 weeks gestation. Once your infant is born, he will seek out the snug environment he experienced in utero. To understand the importance of containment to your premie, watch as he lies in his incubator. The nurse may place him in the middle of his bed. But as he quiets down, he will begin a series of tiny movements that eventually scoot him into one of the corners of the incubator.

You may arrive one day to find your infant scrunched up against a wall or corner of the crib with the sole of one foot in contact with the incubator wall. This is distressing to his nurse because she knows that he can lose body heat through the incubator wall. So she moves him back to the middle of the crib, only to find him in his protected, contained corner again the next time she comes to check on him.

Nestled into that corner, your baby is seeking the confinement he had experienced in the womb. He feels safest and most comfortable when up against a boundary. If you watch him closely, you'll note that he's usually sleeping deeply when he settles into that position. (You'll find instructions on how to create a snug, contained environment for your premie during your absence in Chapter 13, "Shaping the Intensive Care Nursery Experience.")

Containment is also an effective way to prevent inappropriate sensory input. It decreases your infant's perception of

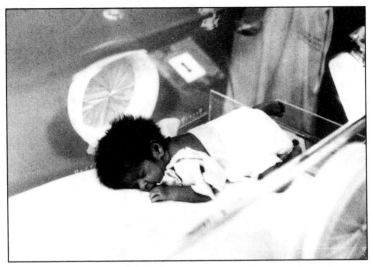

This baby has scooted down into one corner of her incubator. Notice one foot up against the wall.

environmental events. When he's contained, he experiences less airflow around him. A change in airflow or temperature alters your baby's breathing rate and can cause heat loss through convection or evaporation. When he's contained, he's not at the mercy of startle behaviors, which eat up calories. Containment also seems to cut out some of the sounds of the intensive care unit. It is well known that clothing and other swaddling materials such as receiving blankets decrease activity and calm babies.

In Kangaroo Care, you provide containment by placing your infant between your engorged breasts, holding him up against your chest, and putting a covering over his back. Mothers often put one hand on the baby's head and the other on his back.

Flexion is also an element of containment. Because of the limited space within the womb, a fetus's legs must be bent at the knees and his arms must be bent at the elbows. A premature infant is too weak to flex his muscles in order to maintain the fetal position of his own accord; he may lie helplessly in his incubator with arms and legs splayed in extension.

As you can imagine, babies lose heat in this open position,

particularly through those areas where the arteries are closest to the skin: the crook of the arm, the groin, the back of the knee. When your premie straightens his arm, leg, or knee, he exposes these areas to the air.

Such a spread-out posture adversely affects the development of good muscle tone and neuromuscular maturation as well. Research has shown that the flexed position helps speed the maturation of your infant's nerve cells, which can eventually enhance his coordination and development.

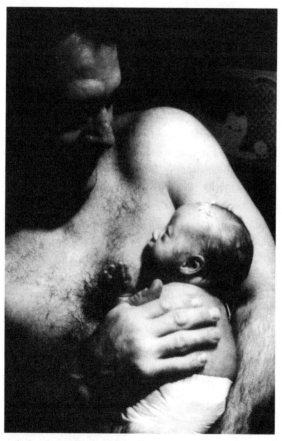

A baby contained on her father's chest with her legs and arms in flexion.

Flexion is reinforced during Kangaroo Care. When you bend your premie's arms and legs, you cut off the exposure of his arteries to the cold air. In so doing, you have not only effectively protected the arteries but have also reduced by half the surface area from which heat can be lost to the air. (In Chapter 10, "Before, During, and After Kangaroo Care," I will show you how to keep your baby in flexion.)

## WHY KANGAROO CARE WORKS FOR FATHERS

Well, you may be thinking, that's all well and good for mothers. But how does Kangaroo Care work for fathers? After all, babies haven't been in their fathers' wombs, have they?

Despite the fact that fetuses have not spent any time in their fathers' bodies, a male's body can provide many of the comforts that a female's can. The continuous quality of the heartbeat, the rocking associated with breathing, and the father's warmth console and quiet the infant. As early as 1913, scientists realized that a baby's heart and breathing rates grew more regular when sounds were presented continuously for at least five minutes. These repetitive sounds quieted babies more effectively than silence.

And, although fathers don't have large, soft breasts with which to envelop their premies, they still provide their own type of containment during Kangaroo Care. Fathers have a firm and consoling type of touch, which is easier to experience than to explain. Try this little experiment: Sit in a chair with a man on one side of you and a woman on the other, and ask each to place a hand on your shoulder at the same time. You will feel the relatively greater pressure exerted by the man's hand, and his touch will feel firm even though it's gentle.

When a father holds his child during Kangaroo Care, he takes advantage of his larger hands. He puts both around his infant's back and essentially engulfs her with his warm, firm but gentle touch. I believe that this protective act also contributes to the success of Kangaroo Care. You'll find more on a father's role in Chapter 12, "Especially for Dad."

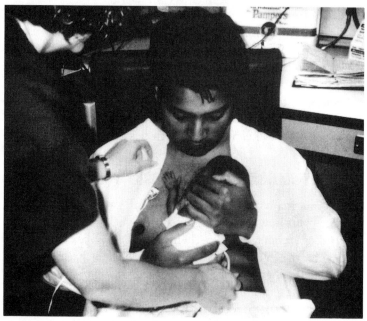

A father's encompassing hands protect, quiet, and warm his child.

## KANGAROO CARE PROTECTS PREMIES

In the 1980s, as advances in medical technology enhanced care-givers' ability to keep premies alive and to save increasingly younger babies, the number of premies who entered the intensive care nurseries grew dramatically. Many hospitals felt it necessary to remodel their units to accommodate the surge of premature infants.

Although the new design accommodated large numbers of babies and allowed easy access to the cribs, it also exposed each and every infant to all of the noxious elements of the environment.

Soon medical and nursing staffs realized that the commotion was less than optimal, for this environment was creating so much infant stress that babies were losing sleep. Researchers have found that premies do much better in semi-isolation. Smaller, more isolated rooms have been found to promote better and faster recovery because they minimize many of the deleterious elements of the intensive care unit.

Kangaroo Care provides the advantages of an individualized environment. As you hold your infant between your breasts, you shield him from drafty air currents. The lighting is softer, and you protect your baby from glare. This is a quiet time. Often nurses consolidate treatment so as not to disturb the infant's sleep. Your baby sleeps with one ear up against your chest, directed toward your heartbeat. One ear is exposed to NICU noises, but I believe that babies shut out these irritating sounds because they fall so deeply into slumber.

## THE CONTRIBUTION OF THE PRONE POSITION

During Kangaroo Care, parents hold the baby chest-to-chest, in an upright prone position. This position has many advantages to your premie. Babies held prone and upright:

• Sleep deeper and longer
• Have decreased energy needs
• Tolerate better the noises and activity around them
• Regurgitate less

If an infant is flat on his back he will be neither well flexed nor contained. His arms and legs will be spread out and at the mercy of atmospheric pressure. Look at a small, really sick infant. He must lie on his back so we can keep him well ventilated. You'll notice that he's pretty well flattened out. It would be difficult for this baby to bring arms and legs over his body to flex them.

When we put that same baby in Kangaroo Care in the upright prone position (even with ventilator), we can turn down the oxygen concentration and the ventilatory control because he requires less oxygen pressure and volume and fewer breathing assists. (Perhaps his chest wall relaxes and allows the air to come in with less resistance and a better volume.)

Bear in mind, however, that research about ventilator

babies in Kangaroo Care is extremely limited, so it's hard to draw conclusions. Clinical observations with ventilated babies show, though, that there is improvement, and if Kangaroo Care is practiced with someone who is closely monitoring the infant's condition, it can continue as long as there's no harm to the infant.

Finally, the upright prone position also contributes to a premie retaining a rounded head. The bones of the premie's head are still quite malleable and susceptible to pressure. When a baby is in an incubator, constant pressure is exerted against the side or back of the skull. He therefore runs the risk of having an elongated or flattened head. This can cause a child social embarrassment as he grows older, since the condition can persist through late adolescence and even into adulthood.

Nurses use waterbeds, air cushions, and frequent position changes to counteract the constant pressure on the skull. The prone position also provides an opportunity for the infant to put weight and pressure on a different part of his skull.

## KANGAROO CARE EMPOWERS PREMIES

Across all the gestational ages and medical conditions, individual differences in temperament, and likes and dislikes, Kangaroo Care seems to have universal appeal. Kangaroo Care babies have their mothers right there to respond to them. When the babies readjust their position, mothers spontaneously and unconsciously help that adjustment. The interplay gives mothers a chance to express their natural maternal feelings. Babies really respond to and enjoy a mother's loving touch.

I believe that preterm babies become empowered during Kangaroo Care. They have gained an ability to influence their mothers, demonstrate their sucking ability, and fall asleep. Just like adults, babies sleep best when they feel safe. Kangaroo Care is a pleasurable experience for them that evokes their feelings of security. Held firmly and warmly in their parents' embrace, the premies' life has returned—if only temporarily—to what it used to be.

# 8

# Is Your Baby Eligible for Kangaroo Care?

During one of my visits to Kadlec Medical Center in Richland, Washington, my research team gained permission to try Kangaroo Care on a very small ventilator baby. Graham had been born at 30 weeks postconception and weighed just over 1,000 grams (about 2 pounds) at birth. We watched this little boy for an hour to get baseline readings on his heart, breathing, temperature, and other vital signs as he lay in his radiant warmer.

Poor little Graham was agitated and irritable! We kept having to stabilize his head and contain his arms. The nurse put her hand on his head to calm him to little avail; Graham was a typical ventilator baby who was coping poorly with all that was happening to him.

We brought Graham's mother in and sat her down, preparing her for her first Kangaroo Care session. It took us a long time—nearly ten minutes—to remove Graham from the radiant warmer and stabilize him and all of his equipment on his mother's chest. But almost immediately, this infant calmed and fell asleep. We monitored him for an hour.

When we put Graham back in his crib, he grimaced in a silent cry. The ventilator tube prevented him from making any noise, but we could see that he was really complaining. His situation was lousy! Carol, his nurse, commented, "Graham seems just as irritable as he was before the Kangaroo Care session."

"That may be true," I replied, "but his unhappiness now doesn't mean that Kangaroo Care didn't help him. He enjoyed an hour of calm and relaxed sleep and that's worth a lot."

I had been so busy with Graham that I hadn't looked around to see who else was in the nursery. It was a typical day at Kadlec: Five other infants filled the beds in the NICU. But now the mother of one of the other babies approached us as we were assessing Graham's post–Kangaroo Care state.

"My infant is irritable, too," she said. "Is that really bad for her?"

"We'd like her to save her energy for growth," Joan, another nurse, replied.

"Well, I saw how calm and relaxed this baby was while he was lying with his mother," she said, pointing to Graham. "I want to do that with my baby, too."

"We'd love to get you involved in Kangaroo Care," I replied. "But since this procedure is so new, we first have to make sure your infant is eligible."

## IS MY BABY READY?

This is no simple matter. Eligibility for Kangaroo Care depends on many factors. Birthweight alone cannot predict which babies are ready for this treatment. I have observed a tiny baby born at 800 grams (just under 2 pounds) who within two weeks was eligible for Kangaroo Care because new lung surfactant therapies (lubricants which help prevent the lungs from collapsing) helped him to breathe on his own better and sooner. On the other hand, I've also seen a 2,500-gram infant (about 5½ pounds) who was so very sick that his many tubes and round-the-clock care prevented him from being positioned in Kangaroo Care.

I should point out here that there has been very little research on using Kangaroo Care with babies under 1,000 grams. In fact, to date only one study has been performed with babies weighing between 1,000 and 1,500 grams. As the use of artificial surfactant increases and becomes more cost effective, however, babies will be better able to tolerate the movements needed to get them in and out of Kangaroo Care and so will be kangarooed sooner.

In general, though, a weight greater than 1,500 grams is usually a green light to begin Kangaroo Care if it occurs in combination with the following other factors:

- The infant's gestational age is at least 28 weeks or his postconceptional age is at least 30 weeks. (*Postconceptional* age refers to weeks in the womb plus out of the womb as opposed to *gestational age*, which refers to only the number of weeks in the womb.)
- He is on stable ventilator settings.
- He is being cared for in an incubator or open-air crib.
- The dosages of his medications have stabilized.

If your baby is under the radiant warmer, he may not yet be a good candidate. The use of this warming unit indicates that he is still quite sick. He may require so many procedures and so much medical attention to maintain life—minute-by-minute interventions—that it may be detrimental to his health and well-being to lift him off the radiant warmer and place him in Kangaroo Care. Given the state of research, I believe it is best to wait until your infant is ready for transfer to an incubator before beginning Kangaroo Care.

Once your baby is in the incubator, he will stay there until he has demonstrated that he can maintain his body temperature, he can consistently take in food and gain weight (15 to 20 grams per day for 3 to 5 days), and he is no longer in need of oxygen supplementation. At this point he will be transferred to an open-air crib. This often occurs between 1,300 and 1,800 grams weight or after a baby is at least 7 days old if his birthweight was 1,500 grams or less.

Most likely you and your infant will start Kangaroo Care

while he's in the incubator. You should be well acquainted with the Kangaroo Care routine by the time he is transferred to an open-air crib.

## USING APGAR SCORES

To decide if your child is eligible for Kangaroo Care at birth, you may use his 5-minute APGAR score. The APGAR helps the health team to determine if your infant needs medical assistance 1 minute and then 5 minutes after birth. Actually, it's a survey of five important factors that help determine the health of the baby:

1. *Appearance:* If your child is pale or blue, he would get a low score for appearance. If he's pink, he would get a high score. Skin color is the most sensitive marker of oxygen saturation immediately after birth.

2. *Pulse:* A heart rate of 120 to 160 beats per minute is good. Less than 100 beats per minute would bring a low score.

3. *Grimace:* How does your baby respond to the discomforts of being born? Does he squint in bright lights and startle at being touched? He would convey his irritability with a grimace. Immediately after birth, crying is a positive reaction. It means that your newborn's central nervous system has responded to his environment. The absence of a grimace would bring a low score.

4. *Activity level:* The health staff will test the tone of your infant's arms and legs by stretching them out and letting them go. If they drop limply, the score would be low. If your child moves them deliberately, then he would get a high score.

5. *Respiratory rate:* Breathing at the normal rate of 35–50 breaths per minute would bring a high score. A crying baby is breathing well and is therefore reassuring. A weak or poor cry would bring a low score.

The lowest score for each of these criteria is 0. The highest score is 2. A baby with an APGAR of 10 would be quite healthy and strong.

The APGAR scale can be used to judge if your premie is ready for Kangaroo Care. A conservative guide would be:

**APGAR of 9–10.** This is a very healthy premie. He can start Kangaroo Care immediately.

**APGAR of 7–8.** A healthy baby. He can probably start Kangaroo Care within the next two days, if not within the first 2 hours of birth.

**APGAR of 5–6.** You may need to wait three to five days before beginning Kangaroo Care.

**APGAR of 0–4.** The medical staff will be so involved in helping this child, you probably won't be able to start Kangaroo Care for seven days or more.

## REQUIREMENTS FOR SICKER BABIES

If your hospital is willing to try Kangaroo Care on your younger, smaller, and sicker baby and has experience with such Kangaroo Care, the following guidelines may be helpful:

1. At birth, the infant must have had a 5-minute APGAR of 5 or more.

2. The baby is a minimum of 28 weeks gestational age and 30 weeks postconceptional age.

3. The infant is on stable ventilator settings. Over the previous 12 hours his care-givers have not had to change the settings to accommodate fluctuations in the infant.

4. The premie's umbilical artery catheter or chest tubes have been removed (or were never required). As I explained in Chapter 4, this catheter goes into the baby's umbilical cord. When you place your baby on your chest, the catheter can press into his abdomen, which can cause it to be obstructed or create false readings. Chest tubes are very fragile and are likely to become dislodged during Kangaroo Care.

5. The infant may be receiving total parenteral feeding (all nutrients are coming in through his blood vessels, as explained in Chapter 4) if the percutaneous line enters his skin at the

crook of the arm. Kangaroo Care should not be attempted if this line comes in at the shoulder, since it can get dislodged more easily than one placed in the arm.

6. The baby may have IVs if they are secure. The security of the scalp vein IVs must be carefully ascertained before Kangaroo Care, again because of the possibility that they may dislodge.

7. The premie may be on medications such as theophylline (regulates breathing) and dexamethasone (promotes lung maturity) if the previous two doses have been the same. If the medical staff is anticipating weaning the child from either of these two drugs during the planned Kangaroo Care session, be sure that the nurses observe vigilantly to determine how he is adapting to the weaning. If you are to use Kangaroo Care while your child is actually being weaned from these medications, plan your session between doses rather than right before a dose is due.

8. Any baby who is on a vasopressor medication (to regulate blood pressure) should not be placed in Kangaroo Care. The upright and relaxed position can alter the blood pressure, thereby changing medication needs.

9. The baby may be receiving oxygen by a cannula, a mask, or "blow-by," but the amount of oxygen required must be relatively stable.

10. The baby may have a grade 1 or 2 *intraventricular hemorrhage* but not a grade 3 or 4, as diagnosed by ultrasound. Intraventricular hemorrhage refers to bleeding into the brain as a result of blood pressure changes within the brain or a change in oxygen level. The lower the grade, the less extensive the bleeding and the better the infant's central nervous system control. A baby with moderate or severe bleeding would be too sick to participate in Kangaroo Care.

11. If your baby is not allowed any food by mouth (in medical jargon, *NPO*) he may still try to go to the breast during Kangaroo Care. (After all, he can't read the doctor's orders!) You will need to get specific instruction as to whether you can allow him to breastfeed. If that is out of the question, you can allow him to suck on your finger instead.

# MINIMAL HANDLING

"I'm a *minimal handling baby*." You may find this sign hung on your infant's warmer, incubator, or crib. Minimal handling is a direction designed to tell the nursing and medical staff that a baby doesn't tolerate well frequent *medical touching*. This does not mean that you should restrict social handling to a minimum; it refers only to medical touch, which, unfortunately, comprises up to 90 percent of the touching that your baby receives each day.

Medical touching is sporadic. The nurse may turn your baby's head, move his leg, or stick his foot. It's intermittent. Babies, especially small ones, react to this type of touch with a decrease of oxygen in the blood. In fact, this type of touch is associated with the onset of premies' low oxygen levels 75 percent of the time. On the other hand, loving touch that contains the baby, like placing your hand on his leg and leaving it there or holding him in Kangaroo Care, does not reduce the oxygen level.

If your baby has a minimal handling sign on his crib, the first thing you should do is ask the nurse:

1. What kind of touch is my baby responding poorly to at this time?
2. Would you monitor my baby as I place my hand on his leg?

You'll be providing a continuous form of touch. Watch your baby's response as your touch stretches over two to three minutes. If he tolerates your social touch without dramatic change in the physiological signs, then he is a candidate for Kangaroo Care.

The minimal handling sign essentially tells the staff to consolidate treatments, so the baby gets all the upsetting touch at one time, and to watch the baby closely, to recognize the effect that medical handling is having. The consolidation of care is believed to promote a baby's ability to recover from the effects of handling.

## ASK THE NURSE OR DOCTOR

When you're eager to start, it can be difficult to have to wait to do Kangaroo Care or any other type of cuddling. Remember that the staff have your baby's health as their number one priority and make decisions most suited to your baby's needs at the moment. But premies' needs change frequently. They can change from week to week, day to day, and even hour to hour. Remind the staff that you're willing to engage in Kangaroo Care if it can help your baby; and when you've seen the signs of readiness that we've indicated, discuss them with your doctor or primary nurse. Remember, they have your interests in mind too.

# PART TWO

# How to Kangaroo Your Premie

# 9

# The Best Times to Use Kangaroo Care

Kangaroo Care is most effective when carried out at the appropriate moment. You must consider several factors, including:

- Your baby's feeding intervals
- The treatments planned for the day
- Your baby's day-night cycling and diurnal rhythms

Let's look at these factors in more detail.

## YOUR BABY'S FEEDING INTERVALS

The timing of your Kangaroo Care session may depend on whether your premie is a gavage-fed or nippling baby. (See Chapter 4, "Life in the Neonatal Intensive Care Unit.") In general, many parents find it best to begin Kangaroo Care just after their baby's scheduled feeding. The procedure can be especially helpful at this time because it keeps the infant in a more upright position than he would be in the incubator. Being slightly inclined can facilitate the digestion of the food. Since your infant's digestive tract is still somewhat immature, the effects of gravity will help to keep his food down.

If you put your baby in Kangaroo Care shortly before a scheduled feeding, the food should be given while he remains in Kangaroo Care, especially if he is receiving his nutrition through a gavage tube. Your infant's relaxation will enable the milk or formula to be taken in less time in many instances. The Kangaroo Care position is believed to create less muscle resistance to the feed.

If your baby is allowed to nipple (suckle), you may want to begin Kangaroo Care an hour or two before feeding. That will enable your premie to rest sufficiently in order to build up the strength to suck well. (Breastfeeding during Kangaroo Care is covered in Chapter 11.) But remember that many babies fall so deeply asleep during Kangaroo Care, you may have difficulty arousing yours at the time of the feeding. If this happens, your premie is telling you that Kangaroo Care should continue for a little bit longer—at least until he awakens spontaneously.

If your premie *must* be fed at an appointed time, then you may want to try the following two approaches to awaken him:

1. Lift him slightly from your chest for a few moments so a little bit of air circulates between him and your chest. Cool air frequently awakens babies.

2. Position him with his head in one of your hands and his back supported in the other so that you can see his face. Gently raise and lower him until he starts to open his eyes. Then gently call his name until the eyes open fully.

It can sometimes take five minutes or more and repeated attempts to rouse a baby out of the deep sleep he enjoys during Kangaroo Care.

If you cannot organize your arrival around a feeding time, remember that whenever you get there, Kangaroo Care will be a beneficial experience for you and your child.

## TREATMENTS PLANNED FOR THE DAY

If you know that your baby is scheduled to have x-rays taken or if he's about to receive an eye examination, it's often helpful to begin Kangaroo Care as soon as the treatment is over. Or if you know that your baby needs an IV and the intensive care unit staff is comfortable with the idea, you may suggest that you hold the baby in Kangaroo Care while the nurses get the IV in place. Kangaroo Care will help calm your infant and enable him to rest comfortably after the disruption. Remember that ideally Kangaroo Care should continue for at least an hour, so squeezing it between treatments for which your infant would have to be removed may be frustrating to the baby and you.

Benefits from Kangaroo Care have been derived from as little as ten minutes of holding, but because premies have such a great need for good quantities of sleep, it's better that they remain in the Kangaroo Care position for at least an hour. This, however, is not written in stone. I don't want you to think that if you can't kangaroo for an hour you shouldn't attempt it at all. Kangaroo Care is not a time-locked intervention any more than holding any other child is. Just bear in mind that more is better than less.

## YOUR BABY'S DIURNAL RHYTHM

One of the goals of developmental care for a premature baby is to help him establish day-night cycling: to be more awake and alert in the daytime hours and to be sleeping in the evening hours. Not only will that help him become adjusted to the ebb and flow of activity within your home, but it will also help you get much needed sleep during your infant's first few months of life.

Our research has shown that in the period after Kangaroo Care, the babies generally sleep better than in the period before Kangaroo Care. So kangarooing in the evening hours may help your baby to sleep for longer periods throughout the night. Over repeated experiences, it may help him get into a pattern of day-night cycling.

You may wish to visit the NICU between the hours of 7:00 P.M. and 9:00 P.M. to hold your baby. This accommodates work and babysitting schedules and can help your premie become accustomed to sleeping more in the night hours.

Finding the time to engage in Kangaroo Care will depend on your schedule and your child's needs. But whenever you choose to do Kangaroo Care, just bear in mind that you are providing your infant with the loving care that will help him to recover from the effects of his prematurity more quickly and successfully.

# 10

# Before, During, and After Kangaroo Care

The moment has arrived. You're about to begin Kangaroo Care. This chapter will show you what to expect and what to do before, during, and after your session.

## GET YOURSELF READY

Before you begin holding your premie, it's best to be prepared. Be sure to empty your bladder before entering the nursery. You won't want to disturb your infant's comfortable sleep with your own toileting needs. Also, if you're likely to engage in Kangaroo Care around mealtime, you would be wise to eat prior to your session. A growling stomach may not awaken your child, but it may render the session less than comfortable for you. Besides, you may decide to spend more time in Kangaroo Care than you had originally planned. Being well-fed yourself will permit you to extend your session, if you so desire.

Make certain that you're healthy. If you're coughing or suffering from a cold or flu, gastrointestinal upset, or fever, postpone your session until you're absolutely well. Your baby will have a natural immunity to your germs, especially if you're breastfeeding, but other infants in the NICU won't. It's best to protect them from infection when they are so fragile.

## CONTROLLING THE HOSPITAL ENVIRONMENT

Make sure that the following conditions are established before you begin Kangaroo Care.

*ROOM TEMPERATURE*

Most hospital nurseries keep the temperature at about 70° to 72° Fahrenheit, and this is just right. But if you live in a warm climate, the intensive care unit may be air-conditioned. In that case, you might want to consider where you're sitting with your baby. Avoid placing yourselves right under the air conditioner vent or, by the same token, next to a window that can become very hot in the afternoon sun.

Research has shown that even when the neonatal intensive care unit is 50° Fahrenheit, babies will be warm enough in Kangaroo Care. But why press the issue? Your infant will waste less energy if the room is warmer for him.

By the time a hospital sends your baby home, his body will have the ability to accommodate the normal household temperature of 65° to 68° Fahrenheit. If you're going to practice Kangaroo Care at home, rest assured that your infant will stay warm at that ambient temperature.

*AIRFLOW PATTERN*

This is a little more complicated than it may seem. Many neonatal intensive care units have a controlled airflow pattern and air supply to minimize airborne bacterial infections. When you visit the nursery, stand by your premie's incubator or crib and consciously determine if you can feel air blowing past you. You won't want your baby to be in a draft during Kangaroo Care.

You should also participate in Kangaroo Care away from abrupt or intense airflow changes. Doors that open suddenly can let in a big whoosh of cool air. Very warm intensive care units may have fans or air conditioning running. You'll want to be away from those sources of blowing air and noise. Drafts can potentially cool you and your baby.

## THE RIGHT CHAIR

I used to believe any chair would do for Kangaroo Care, but as I've researched and learned about mothers' comfort, I've changed my mind on this issue. I recommend the following:

- The chair should be a recliner, especially if you're going to be spending an hour or more with your baby or have a very small baby.
- It should have good padding at the back and the seat. Don't be afraid to bring in an extra pillow if the chair provided doesn't have enough padding or lower back support.
- It should have some rocking capabilities and wide armrests that are not too low.
- It should be wide. A narrow chair gives you little room to move about and reposition yourself. Besides, if the seat is ample, the nurses attending your baby can also put small pieces of equipment next to you as you hold your infant.
- A footrest is a must—during the postpartum period, your legs should be supported and not dangling. Sitting for a long time impairs circulation and can promote the formation of blood clots. If the chair doesn't come equipped with a leg and foot extension, use boxes, phone directories, a little stool, or whatever else you can find to get your legs elevated to half the height of the chair.

### COMFORTABLE AND WARM CLOTHING FOR MOTHER

Plan on wearing slacks or a skirt because you'll be taking off your blouse and brassiere and putting on a hospital gown. If your baby is under 1,000 grams at the time of Kangaroo Care, I recommend that you bring with you a medium weight velour jacket that opens in the front. (This will accommodate all the monitor wires that must be positioned. The nurse will thread the wires under your top so that they emerge at the bottom.) You can zip or snap up the jacket once your baby is on your chest.

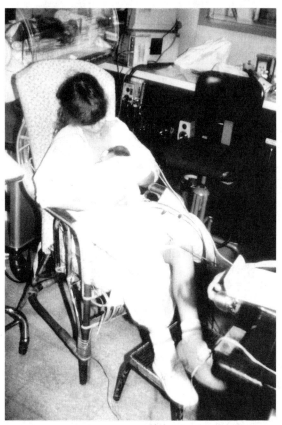
An appropriate chair with footrest.

Our experience has shown us that babies over 1,000 grams will stay adequately warm when covered with a standard hospital receiving blanket folded into fourths and laid across their back. In that case, you can lap the standard hospital gown over your infant's back to conceal your bare chest and further insulate him.

*BREAST PADS*

Women who have been pumping their breasts in anticipation of breastfeeding their premies (see Chapter 11) may experience a significant milk letdown during a Kangaroo Care session. It's wise to come prepared. Bring at least 6 breast pads to each session.

## BABY'S CLOTHING

Your infant must not be totally naked under any circumstances. First, he should be wearing a diaper to protect you from becoming wet. (Moisture will have a cooling effect on your skin and his skin.) The size of the diaper and its positioning will be determined by your baby's size.

A standard premie diaper is often too large on a very small baby. The diaper covers his chest as well as the usual area, and so much coverage would hinder his skin from coming into contact with yours. That would prevent the premie from staying warm, because your body heat would not get through to him.

For very small babies, often a surgical mask works beautifully as a diaper during Kangaroo Care. It can absorb the small amount of urine that these tiny babies produce and provides adequate exposure of your infant's skin to your chest.

If you are using a standard premie diaper with your baby,

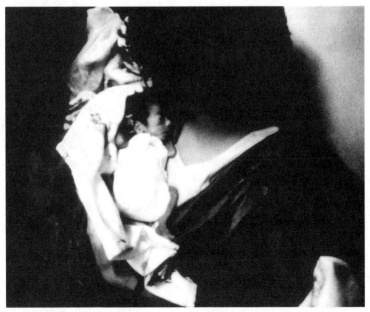

Standard premie diapers can be enormous on a tiny baby.

be sure it's folded down so skin contact can occur from his belly button up.

A baby under 1,500 grams can start Kangaroo Care with a headcap and booties for extra warmth. But don't use the little stockinette caps tied at one end that are so prevalent in delivery rooms. Though less expensive and easier to use, this head covering doesn't retain heat well. If at all possible, purchase a soft, lined woolen hat (available at Abbey Home Health Care retail stores, nationwide). In a research study, these hats were found to have a very good insulation effect and to reduce oxygen consumption by 14.5 percent.

Bigger premies appear to maintain the appropriate body temperature even without a headcap. See below for what to do if your infant becomes too warm during Kangaroo Care.

## BABY BLANKET

A relatively new standard receiving blanket is all you need. Old blankets may be too thin and after repeated washings may lack the pile to insulate your baby adequately and protect him from drafts. If you bring a blanket from home, be sure to wash it after each use.

I start with the blanket folded in fourths, and that usually works perfectly. However, if your baby still seems warm after you've taken off his headcap and booties, you can unfold the blanket once and then twice. In some warm climates, I've removed the blanket altogether and allowed the mothers to simply cover their diapered infants with their hospital gowns. Your baby's abdominal or underarm temperatures are the best measure of his comfort level. When in doubt, ask the nurse to check his temperature.

## SENSE OF PRIVACY

When we first started our investigations into Kangaroo Care, we anticipated that mothers might feel uncomfortable having their chests exposed while their babies were being positioned. If this is your first Kangaroo Care experience, you may want to use a screen. It does take a few minutes to organize and position your baby and his equipment, and a screen can eliminate any unwanted exposure or embarrassment.

By the third session, however, many mothers feel less embarrassment. In general, once mothers become accustomed to the procedure, they don't use the screen, though it is comforting for some to know that it is available, should they need it.

## GET INTO THE RIGHT POSITION

Positioning depends on an infant's maturation and health.

*TINY OR SICK BABIES*

Babies who are limp, flaccid, and weak may be unable to keep their chests expanded during Kangaroo Care. It's hard for these premies to hold their heads erect in an upright position. They may have difficulty breathing under those circumstances, a condition called *obstructive apnea*.

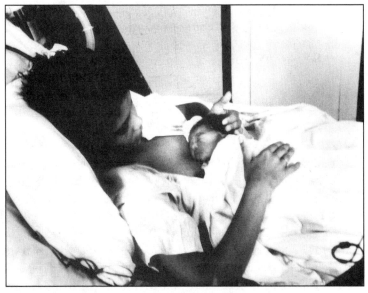

This mother is reclining because her baby is very weak.

If your premie is under 32 weeks and weighs less than 1,500 grams or if she is very sick, you will need to hold her in a more reclined (rather than upright) position. The nurse will help you angle her so that she's resting on one breast or the other. If your infant should bend her head forward as she falls asleep, reposition her head, straightening it to make sure her airway stays open. Watch closely in the first half hour after feeding to avoid gastroesophageal reflux. (See page 117.)

With these babies, you may also want to use a few blankets that have been warmed. Place one up against your chest for a few minutes prior to receiving your baby and leave it in place for the first three to five minutes of Kangaroo Care. This will insure that your skin temperature is quite warm. Place a second one across your infant's back. This is believed to help very small babies recover the temporary temperature loss they may experience during the transfer onto your chest.

## POSITIONING A BABY WHO IS ON A VENTILATOR

Getting your ventilator baby into the proper position requires a bit more preparation and forethought, since you will be dealing with a good deal more equipment. First, ask that two nurses assist you in the transfer of your baby into Kangaroo Care. One will keep all of the equipment and tubes in order, ideally lined up on one side of the body and stabilize your baby's head while the other will actually do the lifting and positioning while holding a blanket over the baby to minimize movement and temperature loss during transfer.

Be sure that you and the nurses have organized the physical set-up for Kangaroo Care before touching your baby. The chair should be close enough to all of the monitoring and treatment equipment such as ventilator tubes and assorted wires and IVs, that these are not pulled or stretched.

Decide with the nurses whether your baby will be transferred into your arms while you're standing beside his bed or seated in the chair. Put yourself in the right spot before receiving your baby. The "equipment" nurse will then line up all of the tubes and wires down one side of your baby's body while the "baby" nurse will place a warmed blanket or diaper over him, containing his arms and legs to prevent any thrashing about (which could dislodge the equipment) during the transfer. As soon as he's in the right position, she will remove the cloth and cover him with the receiving blanket so you can snuggle in together.

If your premie has tubes down her throat for ventilation or respiratory support, her head *must* be turned in one direction or the other so that the ventilator tubes and gadgetry rest on your shoulder. The nurses in the intensive care unit may actually tape these to your shoulder. It's important that a baby in this situation not move her head much because that could dislodge the breathing tube. A semireclined position is probably the most comfortable if your infant has a ventilatory tube.

### POSITIONING AFTER FEEDING

If Kangaroo Care begins right after a meal, it's best to be sitting slightly reclined (at a 60-degree angle) so that your baby's food will stay down in his stomach for the first 30 to 45 minutes. Then you can recline further and get into any position you want. We have not documented at this time any babies having trouble keeping their milk down during Kangaroo Care unless they have *gastroesophageal reflux*.

### POSITIONING A BABY WHO HAS GASTROESOPHAGEAL REFLUX

What does this fancy term mean? *Gastro* refers to the stomach and *esophageal* refers to the esophagus, the pipe carrying the food from the mouth into the stomach. *Reflux* means that food, rather than staying down in the stomach where it belongs, comes back up into the esophagus and sometimes into the mouth. A baby with gastroesophageal reflux runs the risk of choking on his food.

Very small premies with immature muscle tone in the stomach and esophagus can experience this condition usually within 45 minutes of a feeding. So it's important that you remain relatively upright for at least 45 minutes after a feeding if your baby has this problem.

If you're planning to feed your gastroesophageal reflux baby

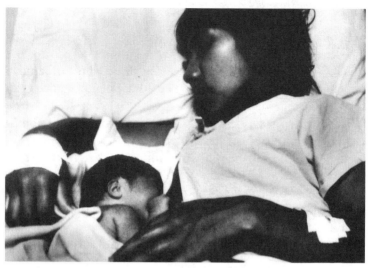

An infant nursing in the side-lying position.

during your Kangaroo Care session, hold him in a side-lying position while he's nursing and then place him upright against your chest once he's done.

When in the upright position, point your gastroesophageal reflux baby's chin slightly upward as if he were sniffing. This keeps the esophagus relatively straight, which is believed to reduce the likelihood of reflux.

*LARGER BABIES*

As your baby grows and matures, you can sit more and more upright with her and she will adjust to that position. By 34 weeks, you can sit almost entirely upright and your baby will be perfectly fine.

## WHAT TO EXPECT DURING KANGAROO CARE

Lois and Allan's baby, Jordan, born at 30 weeks gestational age, was now 35 weeks and doing quite well after having experienced respiratory distress and a major infection. He had been moved into an open-air crib and was capable of sucking from a bottle. He gained weight regularly and had good control over his breathing.

On rounds that morning, Jordan was identified as a good candidate for Kangaroo Care, but his nurses told me that we'd be lucky if we could get his mother in. Lois had three young children at home. Child care was a problem for her, and she had been unable to visit Jordan often. She lived 40 miles from the hospital, and her husband generally took the car. Even if she drove in, she couldn't leave her three preschoolers unsupervised in the waiting room for the two to three hours that our research required.

When I called Lois and offered her the opportunity to participate in my Kangaroo Care study, she asked me if this was a special treatment.

"We're doing a research study," I replied. "Not every baby is eligible to participate. But now that Jordan is doing so well, we thought he could benefit from skin-to-skin contact. If you can get in to see him, it would probably help you in your preparations for taking your son home."

Lois committed to coming in at 6:00 that evening, when Allan could drive her and stay with their other children while she kangarooed Jordan. When she arrived to fill out her papers and sign the consent forms to participate in the study, however, I noticed that her hands were cold and clammy. I surmised that she was nervous.

After Lois had completed the requisite documents, I turned the papers over, sat down beside her, and asked, "Are you concerned about what we're going to be doing?"

Lois looked at me and said, "You know, I have never held my baby."

"Well, you're going to have a chance now," I reassured her. "We'll be with you at all times. If you feel uncomfortable, if you think Jordan is uncomfortable, or if you have to leave, you just let us know, and we'll put him back in his crib."

I escorted Lois into the NICU. She sat down in the chair, we put a screen around her, and began our preparations for Kangaroo Care. We attached a temperature probe (a disk that lies against the skin to measure the skin temperature) with tape to her left breast, about three inches above the nipple, and we unzipped the velour blouse we had given her and separated it slightly without exposing her nipples. As we reached for Jordan, we made sure that all the wires we had attached to measure his heart, breathing, and temperature patterns (for the sake of our study) were going down by his foot. We lifted him and put him on his mother's chest.

Lois did not reach for her baby spontaneously as many mothers do, so I asked her to hold Jordan while I zipped up her blouse. As I inched the zipper to the nape of his neck, I noticed that this premie was beginning the characteristic adjustments all infants make when placed into Kangaroo Care. Initially, he lifted his head and backed it off his mother's chest a bit. He moved it slightly from side to side and eventually decided on the right breast. This he used as a pillow. He turned his head to the left, resting the bulk of his head on the chosen breast. (Smaller babies are so tiny, they usually remain between the breasts.)

Lois grinned broadly. "You know, I think he knows that I'm his mother," she said.

"You're probably right," I confirmed. "You have the same heartbeat he heard in the womb, the same rhythmic breathing, the same voice. Why wouldn't he recognize you?"

After a few moments she exclaimed, "Look! He's moving his fingers. I can feel him moving his fingers and toes."

"Yes," I replied. "Often babies will reach out as they relax and try to nuzzle into your soft body. But that won't last for long. He will settle down very quickly and fall asleep. Just watch."

As I had predicted, soon Jordan's eyelids fluttered open and closed. Within three minutes, he had stopped nuzzling and moving his head. His fingers and toes quieted and he drifted off to sleep.

Jordan remained relatively still for two and a half hours. During this time, Lois did not talk to us. She simply looked at her baby and closed her eyes, opening them every few minutes to reassure herself that he was still there.

Finally she said, "You know, I can feel him breathing. I know he can breathe because I can feel it." She, too, had visibly relaxed.

About a half hour before the end of the Kangaroo Care session, something startling happened. Jordan abruptly awakened, cried hard for about three seconds, and then went right back down into sleep.

This baffled me. Jordan was the first baby ever to cry during my Kangaroo Care research. His was a deliberate, abrupt, lusty wail of extremely short duration. It stopped as quickly and spontaneously as it had begun, and it seemed unrelated to hunger, pain, or boredom, the usual reasons babies cry. Rather, it seemed an unmotivated wail, and one that was perplexing to me, at the very least. I was especially concerned because I knew that Lois had some anxiety about holding her baby. I didn't want her to believe that her embrace had somehow caused her son to cry.

But as I was mulling over these thoughts and concerns, Lois turned to me with tears in her eyes and said, "You don't know how long I have waited to hear my baby cry." She began to weep and kiss her baby.

Lois had interpreted Jordan's cry as a milestone, a source of communication, a behavior commonly expected of normal babies and one that required a strength that previous to this moment he had been unable to muster. For Lois, that cry meant "My baby is going to make it."

Lois had only one thing to say to me as we placed Jordan back into the crib for his feeding and that was "Thank you"— two words that spoke volumes. And I knew that as a result of this positive experience, mother and child were well on their way to a loving and warm relationship.


## KEEPING YOUR INFANT FLEXED

The fetal position (with arms and legs bent and tucked beneath the torso) is the most comforting position for your newborn, since it approximates his posture in the womb. Most likely your baby will begin his Kangaroo Care session in this natural position. As you move about in the chair and as he relaxes, he may straighten out an arm or a leg. If you notice these involuntary movements, simply tuck the protruding limb back under his body.

Keep in mind that when your infant is in a deep sleep, readjusting his position will not awaken him. And eventually, you'll adopt a supportive hold that keeps your baby snuggled up and tucked in!

## HELPING YOUR BABY REGULATE HER TEMPERATURE

Your baby may stretch out an arm or leg from under the blanket or blouse during Kangaroo Care. These behaviors usually are purposeful. They help her cool an extremity so she doesn't become too hot. If you observe this behavior, notice whether your infant is squirming and sweating (usually initially on the forehead). If she isn't, simply put her arm or leg back under your blouse or the blanket.

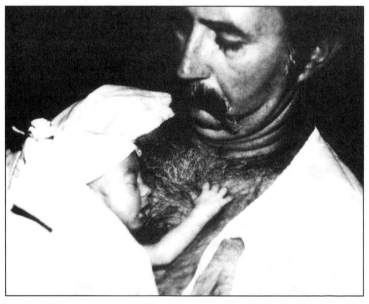

This child is cooling his body by thrusting an arm out of the blanket (thermoregulatory behavior).

If your baby is perspiring, that's a clear sign that she might be getting too hot. In that case, leave the arm or leg where it is and ask the nurse to take her abdominal or underarm temperature. If it reaches 37.4° centigrade (99.4° Fahrenheit), remove the headcap and ask the nurse to reevaluate the temperature in 15 minutes. If your baby is still hot, you can take off the booties.

## TAKING CARE OF YOURSELF

You should also pay attention to your own well-being during Kangaroo Care.

*FANNY FATIGUE*

From my experience, most parents can sit for an hour and a half up to three hours, maximum, before "fanny fatigue" sets in. Although one hour is optimal, because babies deserve this respite, they will get benefits from only 30 minutes of Kangaroo Care. You should not feel guilty if you can only tolerate a shorter session.

*LEGS*

If you're in your first six weeks postpartum, you should stand for 2 to 3 minutes every 60 to 90 minutes to prevent blood clots in the legs. You can walk as far as the monitor wires will allow. Simply hold your baby when you stand. And, remember to keep your legs elevated while you're sitting.

*SLEEP*

Many parents fall asleep with their infants on their chests. This is great! You deserve any opportunity you may have for rest when your baby is in the premature nursery. Take advantage of this peaceful moment of respite and enjoy it with a clear mind. You can feel assured that the nurses are still watching over your infant even as you sleep and kangaroo him.

If you're unable to sleep, you may find it helpful to bring a stereo headset and quietly play music or tapes, especially if you're planning a two- or three-hour session.

*WATER*

Nurseries are hot. You should have plenty of drinking water available before beginning and throughout the Kangaroo Care session, especially if you're breastfeeding.

## KANGAROOING TWINS

If you decide to kangaroo your twins, be sure to hold both of them equally. If not, you may bond to one baby more than to the other! If you're going to hold both babies during the same session, I usually recommend an hour and a half for each, to cut down on your fatigue. It is also possible to kangaroo your children together (one on each breast), but that's best managed if you're lying down. You can also kangaroo one infant while the children's father holds the other. (See Chapter 12, "Especially for Dad.") Just be sure to alternate within the session or on successive days, so that each infant is exposed to the mother's heartbeat.

One mother in Colombia held her twin babies in Kangaroo Care for six hours. When one went to the breast, the other stayed in the Kangaroo Care position; this mother only required the nurse's assistance to reposition her infants for feeding.

Mothers often tell me that they can immediately pick up distinct personality traits in their twins during Kangaroo Care. One twin may prefer the right breast while the other prefers the left. One might be a looker while the other is a sleeper. One might be an active snuggler while the other seems lackadaisical. One might be a barracuda at the breast while the other is a delicate gourmet. And sometimes, mothers comment on how very much alike their twins seem to be. Kangaroo Care becomes an integral part of the claiming and differentiating process.

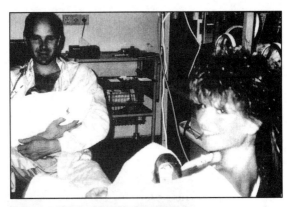

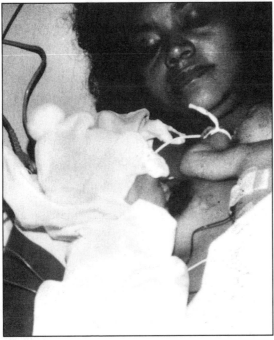

Here are two ways of handling twins taking turns at the breast!

## WHAT TO EXPECT AFTER A KANGAROO CARE SESSION

As the time nears for you to leave your baby in the NICU, he may be fast asleep or even hungry. If deeply asleep, he may continue to slumber during the transition from your chest to incubator or crib. Your standing, his being placed back in his regular bed, and the ministrations necessary to get him adequately clothed or swaddled and nested may all pass unnoticed.

Sometimes babies awaken with all of this activity. Should your infant arouse, stay a little longer if you can. Your soothing words and caresses will soften the transition.

Some babies become mildly agitated, upset, or fussy as they register their displeasure in being moved from the warmth and comfort of their mother's chest. This should not deter you from providing Kangaroo Care. Your baby's temporary unhappiness is most understandable. After all, wouldn't you protest if you were removed from a warm, comforting, familiar environment and thrust into a loud, brightly lit, confusing intensive care unit? In fact, the situation reminds me of the state of pediatric care about 30 years ago.

## "COMPLIANT CHILDREN"

In the past (indeed, in recent memory), parents were severely restricted from visiting their hospitalized children. Sometimes medical personnel allowed visiting hours of as few as 5 or 15 minutes per day. After these brief visits, children became upset. They cried, refused to eat, were irritable and even despondent. The rationale behind the short visits was that children seemed to "do better" when their parents weren't around: They were quiet, compliant, and nondemanding.

Then a psychiatric nurse began looking closely at the situation. She said, "You know, these children aren't quiet and compliant. They're depressed!" She started a study to determine how well the children did if their mothers stayed as long as they wished. She measured health outcomes such as eating, the number of days antibiotics were needed, weight gain, the frequency and severity of complications, and the incidence of behavioral problems (bed-wetting, lack of cooperation with other children or health staff, refusal to engage in treatments).

After careful study, this researcher found that when mothers remain with their children during hospital stays, the youngsters eat better and engage in fewer and shorter regressive behaviors.

This original study, along with the many that followed it, changed pediatric care in America forever. Now mothers are allowed to stay with their hospitalized children all night, and fathers and siblings are allowed to visit the pediatric and maternity wards as often as they wish.

This research and the changes in medical practice hold valuable lessons for Kangaroo Care. Just because babies become upset when their mothers leave does not mean that the mothers shouldn't hold them in the first place! This transient moment of pique is well worth the many benefits the baby derives from Kangaroo Care.

My dream is that in years to come, neonatal intensive care units will be furnished with mothers' beds right next to the incubators or cribs. Mothers would remain with their babies in the hospital. In that way, the nursing staff will be able to perform all medical interventions when the premies are on their mothers' chests. And if mothers are unavailable, certainly fathers can step in.

## YOUR OWN REACTIONS

Although I have never seen this reaction in my own research, Dr. Dyanne Affonso, a professor of family health nursing at the University of California, San Francisco Medical Center, has found that some women, when given the opportunity to provide Kangaroo Care to their infants, become weepy and experience a resurgence of thoughts about the preterm birth experience. They may again feel the grief they felt at the birth and may again ask themselves: "Where did I go wrong?" "Why this baby?" "Could I have prevented this premature birth?"

This reaction may be triggered by the postpartum blues— the normal mood swings and hormonal changes that follow delivery. It is common to have such thoughts. You may need someone to help you identify your feelings: your fears of your infant's death or potential disabilities, your sense of loss at not having a full-term pregnancy and a "Gerber baby," your feelings of responsibility. You may feel a strong need to talk about your emotions and share with other parents who have experienced similar traumatic births.

Today, many hospitals provide support groups run by nurses or social workers for parents with infants in the NICU. Such groups can be extremely helpful; seek one out. And give yourself permission to cry if you want to. You have been through an ordeal. Crying may be a healthy catharsis for you. And, after you have had the opportunity to ventilate your feelings in a safe, supportive atmosphere, you will feel an even stronger attachment to your infant.

# 11

# Breastfeeding During Kangaroo Care

Natalie had a hard time with the arrival of her premie, who was 34-weeks postconception. Postpartum depression coupled with the trauma of the unexpected birth and the demands of her two preschoolers left her in a state of disarray and despair. She had difficulty juggling all of her responsibilities and seemed frustrated and upset whenever she visited her baby, Michael, in the NICU of Kadlec Medical Center in Richland, Washington.

One day, when she came in, my research associate Joan Swinth approached her and asked if she would like to take part in our five-day Kangaroo Care study. Natalie agreed. And as Joan placed Michael on his mother's chest for the first time, she could hear Natalie say softly, "Mommy needed this a lot." This was the beginning of Natalie's adjustment and her ability to handle the premature birth.

After about an hour of Kangaroo Care, Joan instructed Natalie to allow Michael to slide down to her nipple and breastfeed. Although Natalie had been pumping her breast in anticipation of breastfeeding, it was a first for both mother and child. And Michael took to the breast like a fish to water. In fact, he did so well on our Kangaroo Care and breastfeeding regime that he went home from the hospital even before the fifth day of the study!

## WHY BREAST IS BEST

The very best source of nutrition for all babies throughout the first year of life is breastmilk. Breast is best for many reasons:

- It can improve growth by providing the most readily digested and best-suited milk available.
- It contains antibodies we don't know how to get into formula.
- It contains substances such as taurine that foster nerve growth (although increasingly these are being added artificially to formula).
- The rhythmic sucking that occurs during breastfeeding helps regulate heart and breathing patterns and thus promotes better oxygenation of the blood.

## YOUR BREASTMILK IS EVEN MORE SPECIALIZED

It is fascinating to note that the breastmilk of women giving birth to premature babies differs from that of mothers going

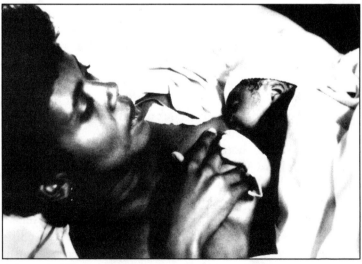

A breastfeeding mother reclines during Kangaroo Care.

full term. Preterm milk has a higher proportion of protein, sodium, and calcium than term breastmilk. This is especially important because a fetus is building bones and muscles until the last four weeks of pregnancy. (During the last month he adds fat.) So breastfeeding your premie will help him catch up to the normal infant in terms of bone mineralization (the bones' density and weight, length, and calcium deposits) and muscle development.

As you can see, your milk is well matched to your premie's needs! But if you are breastfeeding, don't be surprised if your infant is fed formula from time to time. Depending on his condition, he may require supplemental calcium and minerals.

## BREASTFEEDING A PREMIE

Although breastfeeding offers great advantages, the number of women who do it is regrettably low, especially among mothers of premies. In the United States, less than 10 percent of premies' mothers breastfeed. (In the general population, about 33 percent of mothers breastfeed for the first three months.)

Though unfortunate, this is understandable because nursing a premie is not easy. In truth, most premies initially have a hard time breastfeeding for a variety of reasons:

1. *Weak suck.* A premie's suck is usually too weak for her to be able to nourish herself adequately. She may be unable to suck sufficiently to empty the breast. It can take her much longer to suck the milk out than to have milk that's poured into her mouth through a large nipple.

2. *Uncoordinated suck and swallow.* In premies under 34 weeks, the suck-swallow reflex is relatively inefficient, further limiting feeding ability.

3. *Inexperience.* A premie may play around with the nipple, licking it, putting it in her mouth, and holding it without actually latching on. She has to learn what is to be done with the breast. Of course, full-term infants may also need some instruction, but usually a mother can spend two or

three days teaching her child to breastfeed without any grave consequences. A premie, on the other hand, doesn't have that kind of leeway. She must take in calories daily.

4. *Small mouth.* A premie's mouth is so small, her mother's nipple may not even fit into it completely. She may ineffectively pull on the nipple rather than squeezing down on the reservoirs right below the nipple/breast junction (the areola) which would cause the milk to squirt into her mouth.

5. *Nipple confusion.* Until a premie is able to get all of her nutrition from her mother's breast, her food intake will be supplemented with bottle-fed expressed mother's milk or formula. When on the bottle, the infant will experience a flow of milk even if her suck is weak, quite unlike her encounter with the breast.

Because of these difficulties, mothers often become discouraged when trying to breastfeed their premies. You should bear in mind that establishing a breastfeeding routine takes longer than it normally would for a full-term infant. It requires a lot of patience and perseverance on your part—but it is not impossible. With encouragement, support, and many positive experiences, you will be able to breastfeed your premie and, in doing so, cement your relationship with her while giving her a valuable and healthy start on life.

## KANGAROO CARE TO THE RESCUE

Mothers of premies who participate in Kangaroo Care have greater success with breastfeeding. Several studies have found that compared to mothers not involved in Kangaroo Care, 25 to 50 percent more Kangaroo Care mothers are breastfeeding their premies at discharge. Kangaroo Care mothers are able to breastfeed beyond six weeks postdischarge (often when women reenter the work force) with rare supplementation because they produce more milk. In addition, since Kangaroo Care gives them early and more frequent opportunities for breastfeeding, they are more inclined to choose it as the mode of nutrition.

Why does Kangaroo Care encourage breastfeeding? I believe the following factors are at work:

1. *Access to the breast.* Kangaroo Care enables your baby to be a "grazer." Your infant can determine for himself when to eat. He takes in a little bit, digests it, and goes back for seconds, thirds, and more rather than taking the entire feed all at once, every three hours.

2. *Ready source of nutrition.* Your infant doesn't have to cry or wait to be fed. Since he is already at the breast, his hunger needs are easily met.

3. *Your infant is stimulated by the odor of breastmilk.* While lying against your bare chest, your newborn can smell the milk. He may begin rooting around your skin, thinking, "I smell this. Where is it?" In that case, you may slide him down to your nipple, so that he can latch on and suck.

4. *Improved vigor.* Some babies sleep so soundly during Kangaroo Care that once awakened they may become more alert and some will feed more vigorously.

5. *More frequent feedings.* With more breastfeeding experiences, a positive cycle develops: Your infant learns to coordinate breathing, sucking, and swallowing and so becomes a more efficient feeder.

6. *Milk letdown.* As you hold your infant, you become more relaxed. The tension of the premature birth and its consequences melts away. Many women experience a milk letdown shortly after beginning Kangaroo Care.

## THE ADVANTAGES OF BREASTFEEDING DURING KANGAROO CARE

We have found that some babies have more vigor and interest in feeding when they're being held skin-to-skin on their mothers' chests. In fact, most babies go to the breast during Kangaroo Care. It offers early nippling experiences which can facilitate the development of suck and swallow and perhaps speed along the transition from gavage to nipple feedings.

Kangaroo Care may not increase feeding vigor for all babies. Those under 1,100 grams (2 pounds, 7 ounces), seem to have trouble mustering the energy required to feed eagerly. The effort is simply beyond them. If your infant does eat with greater vigor, though, his feeding time shortens.

During Kangaroo Care, your premie can suck on demand and on desire. This is called self-regulatory sucking. He will suck for about a minute and fall asleep, following a pattern of feed and relax, feed and relax. Although he's not getting a big feeding at one time, he takes in continual nutrition as he has the energy for it. Your baby's sucking is under his own control.

This is advantageous for several reasons. Because of this feed-relax pattern, Kangaroo Care is believed to sustain blood glucose levels better than bolus feedings—an all-or-nothing arrangement in which milk is given once every three hours. What's more, it allows your baby to regulate his own feeding schedule. Dr. Peter Gorski, a developmental pediatrician at Northwestern University School of Medicine in Chicago, Illinois, has reported that with self-regulatory sucking, premies

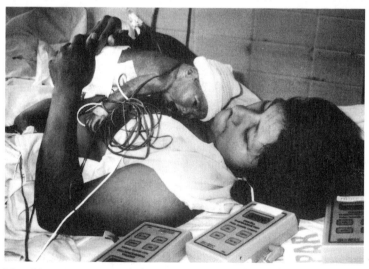

Mouthing movements such as these let you know that your infant wants to nurse.

eat within a shorter time, digest more, regurgitate less, and gain weight faster.

## GETTING STARTED

How do you know if your premie is hungry? He will give you cues. First, he must be awake! He may make mouthing movements or he may even move his head toward your nipple. You may find that he shakes his head from side to side, as if he's saying no. During Kangaroo Care, your infant may even seek out the breast. I have observed infants who have actually crawled up their mothers' abdomens to find their breasts.

When you get these cues, press down on your breast (above the nipple) to express a few drops of milk. This will start the milk flow, soften your nipple so that it can get into your premie's mouth, and provide a small amount of milk to satisfy his immediate hunger. In that way, he won't pull on the nipple and make it sore, which might lessen your desire to nurse!

If this is one of your first few attempts at breastfeeding, be aware that it's a real reward to get any sucking at all. Usually, premies nuzzle, lick, and make skin contact but don't really feed at first. Spend your time cuddling and positioning your baby—and don't feel discouraged!

Sometimes your baby may get on the nipple but may still continue moving his head from side to side. You can help him by stabilizing his head so that he's really latched on. Once that occurs, he'll most likely develop an effective pattern of sucking and breathing.

## SUCKING PATTERNS

Although your young premie may have a relatively weak suck-swallow reflex, you can still begin breastfeeding as early as 30 weeks postconception. Eventually, he will get the hang of it and will suck for several minutes at a time. To get the feeding off to a good start, it may help you to understand your baby's sucking patterns.

During the first minute of feeding, he will begin with a

series of rapid sucks—about two per second. He is not getting much milk. But this nonnutritive sucking helps him build his muscle tone for the all-important nutritive sucking to follow, much like an athlete's warm-ups before competing.

He will pause between these rapid sucks, to catch his breath. Don't coax him back to the breast at this point, allow him to breathe.

By the second minute of feeding, your premie will integrate breathing with sucking. He doesn't need to suck as frequently—one suck per second—and he requires fewer pauses. This is your indication that your milk is flowing heavily and that your infant is breathing while he's eating.

Toward the end of the feeding, your infant may become disorganized in his breathing and sucking. He may pause more frequently, and his sucking pattern may lose its regularity. This is your indication that he's tiring. Don't try to coax him back to the breast; he's letting you know that he has finished his meal.

With time and experience, your milk will let down shortly after your infant begins suckling. This facilitates your baby's feeding. He spends less time sucking, and he concentrates on swallowing and breathing with an occasional burst of sucking to help you along.

## CUES TO WATCH OUT FOR

If at any time your premie demonstrates:

- Choking
- Nasal flaring
- Gasplike breaths
- A decrease in oxygen saturation to 85–88 percent

you must stop feeding him. These signs indicate that the milk flow is too fast and too strong for your infant to control. As a result, he's having trouble breathing.

Depress the nipple with your finger or place your little finger in your baby's mouth to get him off the nipple. Let him take 15 to 30 seconds to reorganize himself and get his breath back before starting again.

You may also notice that while your infant is sucking, he is a grazer or a barracuda, a gourmet or a gourmand. These are all normal feeding patterns. As long as your infant demonstrates to you that he's satisfied (he's quiet, not crying or agitated, and not displaying mouthing movements), allow him his own feeding style.

## REGULATING FLUIDS AND CALORIES

If the NICU nurses are concerned that your baby needs a regulated amount of fluids and calories, they will ask you to express breastmilk (by pump) into a sterile container. They'll measure out the required amount into a Lact-Aid, a presterilized disposable bag suspended between your breasts or over your shoulder. A thin flexible tube attached to the bag is placed against your nipple so that your infant will suck the tube and nipple at the same time.

The Lact-Aid makes sure that your baby learns that his stomach fills when he sucks. Remember, it takes time to build your milk supply, and the use of this little device insures that your baby's nutritional needs are satisfied and he learns how to breastfeed while stimulating your breast to produce milk.

## MAINTAINING YOUR MILK SUPPLY IF YOUR BABY IS NOT READY TO NURSE

With a premature birth, it is possible that you may be eager to breastfeed but your infant is unavailable or unable to do so just yet. In that case, it's important to establish and maintain your milk supply until your child can partake of it.

Be sure to drink eight glasses of water or noncaffeinated liquids daily. Add 600 calories to your prepregnancy diet to replace the calcium and minerals used during the production of milk. Be sure you eat balanced meals.

Establish a regular routine of breast massage and pumping (expressing) soon after your baby's birth. It's important to massage before pumping and feeding. This rhythmic stroking helps unplug breast ducts and allows milk to flow more easily. Ask the nurse to demonstrate the proper massage technique.

It is important to express your milk or pump your breasts with an electric breast pump to make sure each breast is fully emptied. Each breast should be pumped every two to four hours for 10 to 15 minutes. Begin on a low to normal setting. When you're finished collecting the milk, be careful to break the suction on the nipple with your finger. Only pump during waking hours, and use your nights for much needed sleep! Never borrow someone else's manual breast pump or breast shields. These could be contaminated with bacteria.

Pump the milk into the sterile Volufeed containers or plastic bags that the NICU nurses will give you. Label the contain-

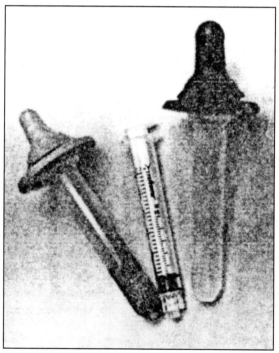

Volufeed containers

ers with name and date and immediately refrigerate the milk for use within 24 hours or freeze it for longer periods. Ideally, though, your baby will consume this milk within 24 hours.

It is inadvisable to rewarm breastmilk slowly at room temperature, since that would promote bacterial growth. Most nurseries use a room temperature water bath to bring stored breastmilk to the proper temperature swiftly. This rewarms the milk more quickly while not exposing it to high temperatures, which could cause the loss of its antibodies. To avoid this loss of antibodies, don't use the microwave or a hot water bath. Of course, milk is best when it's fresh!

Be forewarned that no pump stimulates the breast as well as a baby. In fact, your milk supply may eventually dwindle. Breast massage can help here. It's also useful to look at a picture of your baby or listen to a tape of his sounds to stimulate your milk production while expressing breastmilk. But most important: Don't feel guilty if your milk supply diminishes. It can be built up again. A sparse supply doesn't mean that you can't nurse. When your baby gets on the breast, your body will respond to his needs. The amount of milk you can express by hand doesn't truly reflect how much your baby will suckle.

## ASK FOR HELP

Breastfeeding isn't instinctual. If it were, every woman would be doing it! Rather, it's a learned behavior. You may need help learning how to do it successfully, and hospitals understand this. That's why many intensive care units employ certified lactation consultants. Ask for help if you need it.

You should also ask questions of the NICU staff in order to comply with their breastfeeding routines. Find out:

- How often you should come in to breastfeed.
- If your infant must be a certain weight or gestational age before you can start.
- If the NICU supplies the Volufeeds and sterile containers for the milk. If not, where can you obtain them?

- How fresh the milk should be if you're unavailable during a feeding time so if need be you can plan ahead your pumping routine.
- How long you're allowed to keep breastmilk frozen.
- If milk banking is available. (Your milk is stored for your baby. If there is excess, it may be shared with other babies.) You may or may not wish to participate in a milk bank. Also, make sure donors are screened for infectious diseases.
- If you need to sign a consent form.
- If you can use the hospital pump. If not, where can you rent one for home use?

## BREASTFEEDING IF YOU'VE HAD A CESAREAN

*Oxytocin*, the hormone critical to the milk ejection reflex, triggers the release of milk by causing the muscle cells surrounding the milk sacs to contract. This hormone also causes the muscles of the uterus to contract. This helps the uterus to shrink to its former size and shape and can even feel pleasurable. However, when a preterm infant is delivered by Cesarean section, these uterine contractions can be acutely painful after surgery and can discourage the mother from breastfeeding.

If you have had a C-section, your obstetrician may leave the epidural or intravenous catheter in place during the first 24 hours after delivery. You can administer your own pain medication, as needed, for these contractions.

After the catheter has been removed, it's best to take any oral pain medication after you've breastfed your child so that the medication levels peak before the next feeding. Be sure to confirm with your physician that the medication is appropriate for a breastfeeding mother.

## FATHERS AND BREASTFEEDING

At Memorial Medical Center in Bakersfield, California, ten fathers were given the opportunity to provide their incubator infants with Kangaroo Care (see Chapter 12, "Especially for

Dad"). We were surprised to find that most of the babies in this study started to suck on their fathers' breasts!

We usually assume that the smell of milk attracts an infant to the breast. But here, premies were seeking out a nipple without the usual cue. It is possible that the scent of milk alone does not render the nipple attractive, that an instinctual drive to feed might have caused the babies to go to the male breast. Or, perhaps the visual appearance of the nipple also plays a role.

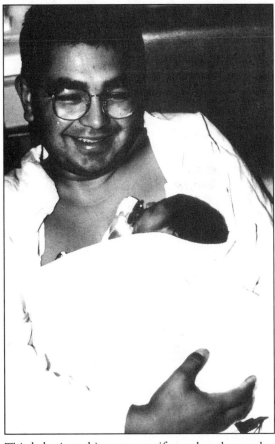

This baby is sucking on a pacifier rather than on her father's breast.

At any rate, one father commented on his infant's surprising attempts at breastfeeding when he recorded his impressions of the experience. "Despite his sucking," Barry wrote, "and the 'cuteness' associated with it, I felt no loss at not being able to breastfeed (an old wives' tale I've heard)."

Another father became uncomfortable with his baby's attempts to suckle at his breast. We instructed him to slip a little finger into his premie's mouth to break the suction. We then provided the baby with a pacifier to encourage his nonnutritive sucking.

## NONNUTRITIVE SUCKING

You'll want your baby to have opportunities to suck on her own fingers or on a pacifier when you're not available. According to research in this field, nonnutritive sucking has many benefits for your baby, since it:

- Helps her heart rate stay more normal
- Builds strength in her cheek muscles
- Satisfies a reflex to suck
- Improves oxygenation during tube feedings
- Encourages earlier and more organized sucking patterns
- Enhances weight gain (even though she's taking in same number of calories)
- Promotes earlier and faster feedings
- Encourages earlier discharge from hospital
- Promotes better mental and motor scores at 2 years of age

Nonnutritive sucking is one of the most effective ways to get your baby to be alert so she can look at you and learn to know who you are!

# 12

# Especially for Dad: Paternal Kangaroo Care

I first tried Kangaroo Care with a father during a 1988 study at Hollywood Presbyterian Medical Center in Los Angeles. Jim joined his wife Betsy while she was holding their premature baby. Lisa was now 33 weeks postconception and weighed 1,825 grams, about 4 pounds. She had progressed to an open-air crib and was getting ready to go home the following day.

All was going well during Lisa and Betsy's three-hour Kangaroo Care session. The temperature probes on mother and baby showed that Betsy's breast temperature fluctuated while Lisa remained toasty warm.

Jim came in and stood behind us. He watched as we collected data on his baby and wife. A radio engineer, this dad focused on all the indicator needles and readouts on the equipment. "What are all those wires for?" he asked.

"We're watching your infant's temperature," I explained, "to make sure she stays warm. This wire [I indicated the one on Betsy's breast] measures your wife's skin temperature as it responds to Lisa's."

Then Betsy looked up at her husband. "Jim," she said, her eyes shining with excitement, "this is just the most wonderful thing I have ever experienced! I've finally had a chance to hold Lisa."

Jim turned to me and said simply, "Now it's my turn to kangaroo."

Although I wanted to accommodate this dad's request, I had some trepidations. Jim was a big, trim man without body fat padding across his flat chest. Basically, he had no breasts to prevent drafts around the baby. What's more, I could see that my special velour blouse was never going to fit around his brawny shoulders. I had no confidence that he would be able to keep Lisa warm, and I certainly didn't want a baby to have problems during one of my first studies in Kangaroo Care.

Reluctantly I replied, "It's not possible."

But Jim wouldn't take "No" for an answer. "I have every right in the world to hold my baby, too," he said adamantly. "I'm going to ask the doctor to let me do it."

So the neonatologist was summoned, and he said that Jim could hold his daughter in Kangaroo Care but that he himself would stay with us to make sure Lisa did not develop cold stress if Jim proved incapable of warming her sufficiently.

Jim was wearing a thin cotton shirt. We unbuttoned it and placed Lisa on his chest. His big hands engulfed the tiny baby. Then we draped a blanket across his hands and Lisa's back. Jim sat in the chair his wife had been in, while we anxiously watched all the monitors.

As Jim observed my anxious expression, he said, "Don't worry. I'm keeping this baby warm. I can feel my skin opening up and giving warmth to her. She's not going to get cold."

Jim was right. His infant didn't get cold, despite my concerns. After he had completed Kangaroo Care for one hour, Jim said, "It was really rewarding to see Lisa do well. She's been through so much. I can't wait to get her home."

A second opportunity to try Kangaroo Care with dads arose at Kadlec Medical Center when Dr. Anderson and I were visiting the study on incubator babies experiencing Kangaroo Care.

Kathy had completed her Kangaroo Care session with Caroline, who had just come off the ventilator the day before. Kathy had been in frequently to visit her baby and always wanted to hold her. Today her husband Marc was there, too.

When Kathy finished kangarooing, Marc turned to our neonatologist, Dr. Anthony Hadeed, and asked, "May I do it, too?"

Dr. Anderson was enthusiastic about the idea because she had observed fathers successfully engaged in Kangaroo Care with small incubator babies in Europe. We decided to try Kangaroo Care with Marc even though his baby was quite small.

Again, the trial was successful. Marc's tiny incubator baby snuggled into his chest, grabbed on to a tuft of hair, and smiled. We monitored the baby's condition for about an hour, and she did just fine. She stayed warm and contented and only

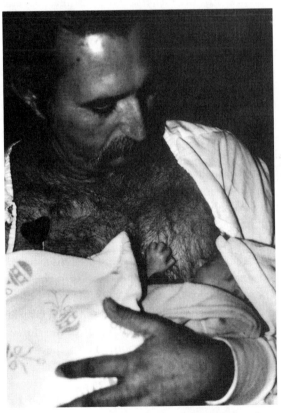

A baby reaches out and grabs his father's hairy chest during Kangaroo Care.

protested when we took her off her father's chest to go back to the incubator.

I had now been fortunate enough to see a father using Kangaroo Care with an incubator and an open-air crib premature. When the opportunities arose for investigating paternal Kangaroo Care in Cali, Colombia, and Bakersfield, California, I was eager to take advantage of them.

## MY RESEARCH WITH FATHERS IN LATIN AMERICA

In 1992, Dr. Robert Hosseini, a member of our research team, went to the Hospital Universitario del Valle, in Cali, Colombia, to coordinate a study on fathers using Kangaroo Care within the first 24 hours after birth.

We took a conservative, wait-and-see approach, since we were uncertain if traditionally macho Latin American men would want to kangaroo their premies. As expected, the study was not without its complications. First of all, because fathers in Colombia are not routinely let off from work when their wives go into labor, many weren't in the waiting room and thus were unavailable to even be asked if they wanted to participate in Kangaroo Care during the first day after birth. Second, when fathers were available, their visits were of short duration. Moreover, fathers in this South American country were unaccustomed to baby care, a task almost always assigned to women. Kangaroo Care was an unusual idea to them, and many wanted time to think about it.

Despite these obstacles, over the course of three months we were successful in finding 11 fathers who came into the hospital and held their babies in Kangaroo Care for two hours.

We asked the men to arrive at the time of their babies' feeding, and while their wives were breastfeeding, the nurses took the fathers to the Kangaroo Care room. There the nurses examined them for any infections, such as upper respiratory or skin infections.

After the fathers got clean bills of health, they scrubbed their chests and arms from top to bottom for three full minutes. (Newborns have a natural immunity to their mother's germs but no such immunity to their father's.) Then the nurses instructed the men to sit in an upright, stationary chair at their wives' bedsides in the Kangaroo Care room.

In each case, we put a clean hospital blanket over the father's lap and handed him the baby, who had just finished feeding. The infant wore diapers, a headcap, and booties. We folded another clean hospital baby blanket in fourths and placed it across the premie's back. The infant was connected to all the requisite physiological monitoring devices (measuring heart rate, breathing rate, breathing pattern, and skin, toe, and core temperatures) so we could see how he adapted to his father's embrace.

And how did the babies fare? Just as they do for their mothers, the infants predominantly slept during Kangaroo Care. They appeared relaxed and comfortable.

Our scientific findings showed that the premies adapted well to this procedure. Their heart rates, respiratory rates, and breathing patterns were clinically normal. They all warmed up. In fact, they may have gotten too warm. It suggested to us that fathers lack the mechanism to regulate their babies' temperatures that mothers seem to have. But this warming was expected because Cali has a tropical climate. The average room temperature is 95° to 100° Fahrenheit, coupled with high humidity.

The fathers acted as most men do when first encountering their premature infants. They talked mostly to their wives and made few attempts to engage the newborn in interaction. Actually, this was quite appropriate because we wanted the infants to sleep. So, these fathers, who for the very first time in their lives were handling babies so young, responded reciprocally to their infants' state: They let sleeping babies sleep.

The fathers' responses to the experience were overwhelmingly positive. One dad observed, "I felt very curious and a little afraid because it was the first time. But the baby kept on sleeping with a lot of love." Another gushed, "I feel very happy to have my baby on my body. This gave me so much joy. I have never felt so much happiness."

## PATERNAL KANGAROO CARE RESEARCH IN THE UNITED STATES

The data coming from the study in Cali, Colombia, showed that we needed to determine if the warming that occurred there is common to paternal Kangaroo Care regardless of climate, so we undertook a second Kangaroo Care study with fathers, this time at Memorial Medical Center in Bakersfield, California.

We observed the babies for 30 minutes in their incubators right after their feeding. We then let their fathers hold them for two hours. Finally, we put the premies back into their incubators for another 30 minutes of observation. We were able to collect data on 10 babies and their fathers using this method.

We watched heart rate, respiratory rate, oxygen levels, breathing pattern, abdominal temperature, toe temperature, and core (internal body) temperature. We also recorded the babies' state minute-by-minute, noting whether they were awake, asleep, crying, active, or inactive.

As we had come to expect, the babies all warmed up, went to sleep, appeared happy, frequently smiled, and even went to their fathers' breasts during Kangaroo Care. And, as we had hoped, there was also a poignant and moving response on the part of the fathers.

## FATHERS' REACTIONS

Kangaroo Care worked its usual magic with the infants in Bakersfield. More than that, it drew fathers into the care of their premies. Novice and experienced fathers alike commented on the positive feelings they had toward their children after Kangaroo Care. "Prior to the experiment," John explained, "I was looking forward to having Daniel at home. Now I can't wait. I don't feel as anxious about holding him, and I don't want to leave him now. Much of my worry regarding my ability to handle him has dissipated. It was a very enjoyable experience, and I actually feel closer to him."

Another dad, commenting on how long it had taken him to develop a relationship with his other children ("All they did was eat and sleep. There was no interaction for me till they were toddlers"), said that after his Kangaroo Care experience he already felt closer to this child than he had to his older two as babies. "There's an increased chance of enjoyment for me early on as compared to the other children," he wrote on his comment sheet. "I see her differently now, better!"

In general, the fathers responded with genuine warmth; their comments indicated that the important bonding process had begun. As one dad explained, "I love the way he slept and appeared comfortable with me." Kangaroo Care may have played a role in cementing the bond between father and baby.

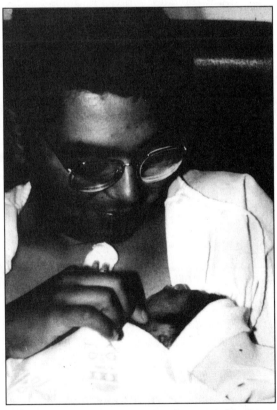

A father lovingly explores his infant with his fingertips during Kangaroo Care.

## FATHERS' CHEST TEMPERATURES

One of our early findings with maternal Kangaroo Care was the mothers' ability to alter their chest temperatures to accommodate their babies' body warmth. To see if fathers were able to do the same, we placed a probe on their chests. We put it on the right side of the chest, so we wouldn't be measuring the heat generated by the heart, but rather the breast temperature.

We learned that all fathers' chest temperatures are higher than the temperatures babies require to keep them from getting cold. But, as we had noted in Colombia, fathers seemed unable to adjust their body temperatures to match their infants' needs. As a result, the babies in Colombia got overwarmed on their fathers' chests. But the babies in the Bakersfield study (where we had a moderate climate and air conditioning) didn't become overwarmed even though their fathers' temperatures were the same as those of the South American fathers.

From this we concluded that the Colombian infants' warming was related to the relatively high room temperature and humidity. We realized that we must be vigilant in our observation of paternal Kangaroo Care in warmer climates. In addition, we needed to implement early on precautions that would prevent overheating.

## WHAT TO DO

Since paternal Kangaroo Care has created positive experiences for fathers and babies, you might want to try it, too. If you do, be sure to adhere to the recommendations and precautions outlined in Chapter 10, "Before, During, and After Kangaroo Care," as well as to the following:

1. Make certain that you're healthy. If you're coughing or suffering from a cold or flu, gastrointestinal upset, or fever, postpone your session until you're absolutely well. (Babies have a natural immunity to their mothers' germs, especially if they're breastfeeding, but not to their fathers'.)

2. Be sure not to overcommit yourself. Two hours seems to

be a father's maximum. An hour to 90 minutes is certainly adequate for a kangaroo visit with your baby.

3. Scrub in. The nurse will instruct you on how to scrub your arms, fingers, hands, neck, shoulders, and chest. This may be crucial for preventing infection, though fathers in Europe only shower and wear clean clothing before kangarooing.

4. Wear clean slacks.

5. You will be given two clean blankets: one to be laid across your lap over your slacks and one to cover the baby's back.

6. When your infant is placed on your chest, be sure the folded blanket covers his back. You may engulf him in your hands and support his head.

7. Don't be afraid to move around and change position once your infant has been handed to you. You can even stand and take a step away from the chair, but be careful of the leads and be sure to support your baby's head against your chest to prevent it from flopping forward and backward. Move around to improve the circulation in your own legs.

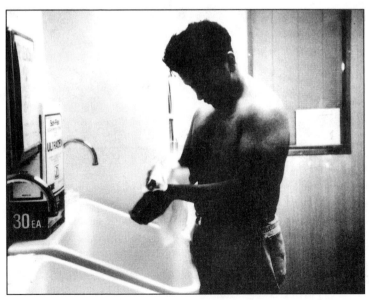

A father scrubs in before practicing Kangaroo Care.

8. Anticipate that your baby may go to your breast. After sucking for a short time, he may learn that your nipple is nonproductive, stop sucking, and fall back to sleep. When and if you are uncomfortable with him sucking on your breast, remove the baby by gently slipping your little finger in his mouth and easing him away from your nipple. Offer a pacifier to satisfy your baby's needs.

9. Be prepared to feel warmth. Babies get warm in Kangaroo Care, and you may be surprised how warm you become. You might wish to have a glass of water nearby.

10. Don't be afraid to talk to others around you. It shouldn't awaken your deeply sleeping baby.

As a result of our research, I can firmly state that fathers are as capable as mothers of giving their babies a reprieve from the environment and protecting them from the overstimulation of the neonatal intensive care unit. The rest is up to you!

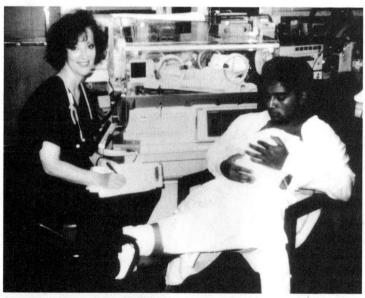

A father fully at ease, providing Kangaroo Care to his newborn while nurse researcher collects data.

# 13

# Shaping the Intensive Care Nursery Experience

As much as you may want to, you can't always be at the NICU with your baby. And the hospital environment, by virtue of the tasks nurses must accomplish, is highly structured and oriented toward routine. It certainly isn't like home! When your baby starts to fall asleep in your own home, you're apt to shut off the phone ringer and lower the shades. When she awakens, you come to her quickly. When she fusses, you hold, feed, or change her. In these ways you are being reciprocal to her needs. You let her sleep when she's sleeping and you interact with her when she's awake.

As I explained in Chapter 4, often the stimulation within the neonatal intensive care unit is nonreciprocal; it occurs irrespective of your premie's needs or ability to handle it. Since nurses and doctors have other patients that will take them away from your baby, *you* are the best person to initiate and continue with individualized, reciprocal care in the NICU.

The first step in the process of reciprocity is understanding your baby's messages (see Chapter 5) and trying to eliminate as fully as possible any activity that produces distress. The second step is to shape the environment within the NICU so that it's the least disruptive and the most comforting to your infant, even in your absence. Your goals should be:

- Protecting your child from the most noxious elements of the environment
- Reducing your infant's agitation
- Promoting your premie's sleep
- Replacing harmful experiences with pleasant ones

The following suggestions will help you modify the environment and contribute individualized care for your premie.

1. *Assess the lights in the environment.* Are there florescent lights? If so, you will need to devise ways to shade your baby. If the lights are not fluorescent, does the intensive care unit have baby-specific lamps? Let the staff know you'd appreciate their using only baby-specific lamps for your infant.

Is your child near the window? The sun provides an extra (and in this instance, unwanted) source of light. You'd want to position your infant so that the light isn't shining in his eyes.

Are the overall lights in the unit on a dimmer switch? Although it may be difficult, try to encourage the staff to install one if none now exists. If the unit is equipped with dimmers, encourage the staff to use them.

If all else fails, you might try covering the incubator with a light-cutting film manufactured by the 3M Company. But do not put sunglasses on your premie. This only distorts his visual acuity. Premies start life with immature visual acuity in the first place; sunglasses only make it worse. And babies won't pay attention to distorted visual images.

2. *Assess the noise level.* Is a radio playing twenty-four hours a day? This is a source of constant auditory stimulation and irritation. The radio should be turned off for at least 20 minutes during each eight-hour shift.

How close is your baby to the entrance and scrub room, the nurses' station, telephones, and stamping machines? These create a lot of additional noise. Ask for your premie to be placed far away from these sources of extraneous high-intensity sounds.

Where is the trash can? Raising and lowering the trash can

lid with a foot lever is loud—110 decibels. Ask the nurse if the lid can be padded or moved to another location. In fact, see to it that as much equipment as possible (especially the incubator lid) is padded to cut down on noise.

Determine when the intercom system is most in use. It's a good idea to schedule naps when the intercom is routinely silent. Ask the personnel to try to give some quiet time to everyone.

3. *Assess the layout of the intensive care unit.* Do you have the option of getting your baby into a two-bed room? A nursery room accommodating four infants is better than one accommodating eight. Research has shown that babies in quiet rooms have more quiet sleep and sucking and less purposeless activity than babies in noisy rooms. In the study, the babies in quiet rooms were actually discharged from the hospital one week earlier than control infants.

4. *Ask about nap time.* Ascertain if you can designate a period as "nap time" for your baby. Ask the nurse when medical and feeding routines involving your baby usually take place. Can you put a little sign on the crib that says, "Please do not disturb me. This is my nap time," when these tasks have been completed? Set up a plan with the nurse for scheduling Kangaroo Care so your premie can nap on your chest.

5. *Establish day-night cycling.* In addition to nap times throughout the day, ask if it's possible for your baby to get some day-night cycling. Often the nurses in the NICU soften noise, dim lights, and encourage sleep between 11:00 P.M. and 6:00 A.M. But you can also help out.

Put a sleep shade over your baby during the night to facilitate his day-night cycling. You can make one from purplish or navy blue fabric. One mother used black fabric printed with little moons and stars. Another sewed a red scarf on top of a blue scarf. Once you've created or purchased the shade, you might want to write or embroider your baby's name on it.

Bring the sleep shade in on your next visit with your premie. When placing it on his incubator, allow it to cover the top and two sides of the crib. But leave open the ends from which the wires emerge. By the way, you can use the sleep shade during your premie's daytime naps, too.

6. *Nesting.* Premies scoot over to the corners of their incubators in their attempt to re-create the containment they had experienced in the womb. (See Chapter 7, "Why Kangaroo Care Works.") Since your infant may be sleeping soundly and breathing evenly when pressing into a corner of his incubator, you may wish to leave him in this position. Simply slip a diaper or blanket between his foot and the incubator wall. This will prevent loss of body heat, and the movement probably won't awaken your baby.

If, on the other hand, the nurses want your baby to remain in the middle of his incubator, you'll need to provide boundaries for him by encircling him with rolled blankets. Surrounding the head seems to be very calming to babies; keeping his sides and feet contained will diminish useless activity and conserve his body heat. Your infant should be nested at all times.

Contain your infant within his incubator between bolsters of fabric that are at least as high as his body. There are various ways of creating these bolsters. You can use: rolled blankets, foam forms, rubber doughnuts, hammocks, a "Neocrate,"

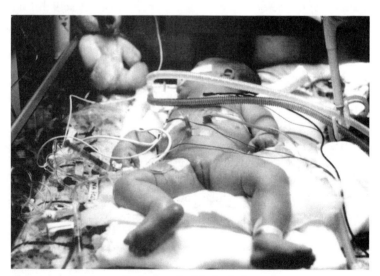

An unnested baby easily loses valuable body heat.

miniature sleeping bags manufactured by Snugli, or bean bags (about the size of your premie) that you've covered with soft fabric.

The hospital's occupational or physical therapist can help you create an appropriate foam nest, addressing your baby's particular needs for flexion and muscle tone development.

A rubber doughnut keeps babies well flexed and well contained. (These are routinely used in the maternity ward for women who have had episiotomies and can be purchased at health care retail stores nationwide.) Dr. Paul Helders, director of neonatal physical therapy at the University of Utrecht, Holland, uses rubber doughnuts and found in a long-term study that babies developed better when positioned in them throughout hospitalization.

Most institutions have water bed mattresses available upon request. These can provide a nest, too. If your baby is on one,

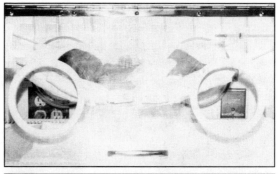

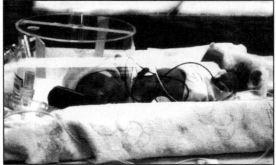

Here are various nesting options: A premie nested in a hammock (top); A blanket roll makes a fine nest (bottom).

he may enjoy several advantages. The water within the mattress is heated to facilitate temperature control, and these mattresses mold more completely to a premie's fragile bones than do conventional mattresses. The use of a water bed, therefore, also reduces the head-flattening that is common in premature babies.

Lambskins are also useful in creating a nest. In some studies, babies on lambskins tend to sleep and eat better and gain weight faster. They seem to nestle in and feel secure. If you use a lambskin, put it under your baby and roll and tape the edges to create a nest. Purchase one meant especially for babies. It should be triple-brushed and guaranteed not to let

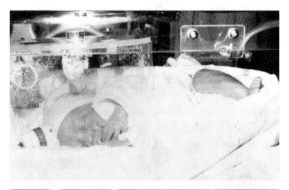

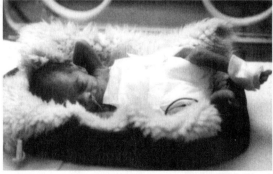

This nest includes foot support (top); A rubber doughnut provides a snug and comfortable nest (bottom).

loose fibers that your baby could inhale. (I recommend the "Lamby" lambskin, available by calling 707-763-4222.)

A headcap is also part of nesting. Your baby should wear one at all times. (See Chapter 10, "Before, During, and After Kangaroo Care," for the best headcaps to use.)

7. *Positioning.* In the womb, your fetus was naturally flexed. In the intensive care nursery, keeping your premie in the flexed position within his incubator helps prevent the loss of his body heat.

Use your nesting equipment to keep your premie's legs and arms flexed. The nest should be close enough to his shoulders to keep his arms in close to his body.

As much as possible, we like to keep the baby's body at *midline* when he's lying on his back—that is, with his head turned to neither the right nor the left. Even if your baby is on a ventilator, the nurses can position the tubing so his head isn't turned to one side. All forms of oxygen can be delivered in this position and will be accompanied by decreases in the blood pressure in the brain.

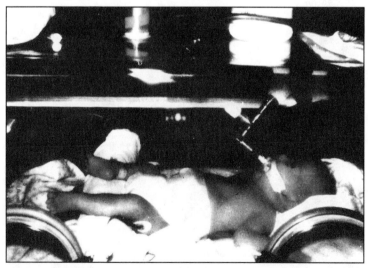

This ventilator baby's tubes are positioned so the head remains at midline.

In general, babies tend to sleep better on their stomachs. The oxygen level in their blood is higher when they're prone than when they're lying on their backs; their airways stay open, and they experience better neuromuscular development, less skin trauma, and less regurgitation.

Even ventilated babies can be placed prone. Sometimes, however, it is difficult for young premies to remain flexed while prone. We lay these infants on a rolled blanket which extends vertically under their chests from breast to hips. This allows their arms to flop down. In such a position, the shoulders, arms, and knees flex naturally.

Recently an association has been made between this position and Sudden Infant Death Syndrome (SIDS), so your institution might be reluctant to place your premie prone. Nonetheless, bear in mind that no one yet knows the cause of SIDS. It has also been correlated with other factors such as low body temperature, sleep disorders, and apnea.

As long as your infant is continuously monitored, I advocate the prone position, because the vigilant observations of the attending nurse and the sophistication and accuracy of contemporary monitoring equipment insure that any life-threatening situation will immediately be recognized and

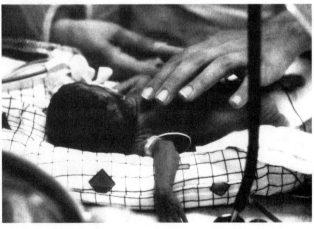

A young premie sleeping prone on a beanbag.

corrected. After all, the purpose of intensive care is to watch your baby intensively. If your infant is not intensely monitored, the use of the prone position should come under the guidance of your health professional.

## A MOTHER BECOMES EMPOWERED; A BABY GETS WELL

Elaine came to one of my community talks on ways to enhance infant development. Her premie, Marla, was born at 28 weeks with multiple medical challenges. After the first week of Marla's hospitalization, Elaine began having problems dealing with the premature birth and her sick child. A high-achieving woman in a pressured industry, Elaine was having trouble accommodating the birth of a tiny premie. Her infant's condition made her feel like a failure. Unfortunately, avoidance became her coping mechanism. She hardly ever visited Marla in the intensive care nursery, and when she did come, she stayed for a relatively short time. This mother was keeping track but she was uninvolved.

Since Elaine was having such a hard time, the nurse caring for her premie recommended that she attend my lecture, which covered information I've shared with you in this book. Fortunately, Elaine took my suggestions to heart. The very next morning, she went back to her baby and started right off by making an assessment of Marla's environment. She found that her incubator was near the unit's centrifuge (where the nurses spin down blood for analysis two or three times a day). She asked that Marla's crib be moved to the other side of the nursery, away from the equipment—and it was.

Next, Elaine decided she was going to modify the light intensity. She began a search for a navy sheet to cover her baby's incubator. Unable to find such an item in the store, she purchased some black fabric and used this as a sleep shade.

When she brought the sleep shade into the nursery, she met with some resistance. Health personnel are used to being able to look over at a baby, as they use the child's color to gauge oxygenation. I advised Elaine to ask the nurses that whenever they didn't need to look frequently at the shade of the skin they simply let Marla sleep in the darkened, womblike environment. If they needed to check the skin color, they could pick up the fabric and check. Although the nurses were reluctant, they also knew that too much light can be damaging to a premie's eyes, so they allowed Elaine to use the shade.

Next, Elaine padded the sides of the incubator by using half-inch foam pads. She placed one at Marla's head, one at her foot, and a third on the side that was away from the nurses' station. For containment and swaddling, she brought a baby comforter that she had converted into a premie "sleeping bag." (She folded the comforter in half lengthwise and sewed together the foot. The second side tied closed—she did not use a zipper because they can be cold.) This worked nicely to keep Marla warm.

Elaine had built a nest for her premie. As a result, she felt closer to her child and more able to mother her. The fact is, when Elaine had been uninvolved, her baby wasn't developing well. But only one week after she had made the changes, the physician in charge called for a care conference to determine what had transpired to cause the reversal in this infant's condition. Marla had started eating, her blood pressure improved dramatically, and her oxygen saturation values were up while the carbon dioxide values dipped. Happily, she showed daily improvement: She became less irritable, slept more, and cried less.

During the conference, the clinical nurse specialist, Ellen Duerr, volunteered the answer. "I know what happened," she explained to the physician. "Elaine went to a conference on how to shape the NICU environment, and it seems to have made all the difference in the world."

Nursery shutdown, reduced lighting, and sleep shades are examples of conditions you can implement or advocate to protect your infant from the stressful NICU environment. Distancing your baby from sudden loud noises and nesting him will reduce his agitation. Day-night cycling, prone position, and nesting all foster better sleep, as does Kangaroo Care. And Kangaroo Care also has the potent role of replacing noxious experiences with pleasant, loving ones.

# 14

# Kangaroo Care at Home

$D$otty went into labor at 34 weeks gestation. When her bag of waters broke and labor continued, the premature birth of her baby was imminent. Chad was born at 2,184 grams (4 pounds, 13 ounces). He was well at birth with APGARs of 8. He went to the NICU mainly for observation.

Because of his excellent status, Dotty was able to hold Chad in Kangaroo Care from the second day of his life. She really enjoyed it; in fact, she had no desire to stop. The afternoon before her son's release she approached me and said, "Dr. Ludington-Hoe, can I continue holding Chad like this at home?"

My response was immediate and emphatic. "Of course," I said with a smile. "It would be the best thing you could do for him!"

"That's great," she replied. "But how should I proceed? Do I have to sit in a chair like I do here? Should I be undressed? And how long should I hold him? I don't want to waste a minute getting started!"

I was delighted to see this young mother's commitment to and enthusiasm for Kangaroo Care because I have found that practicing this simple procedure at home can extend the many gains a premie experiences during hospital-based Kangaroo

Care. The benefits of home Kangaroo Care have been established in several research investigations that have followed the progress of over 4,000 premature babies and their mothers. I was able to answer Dotty's questions based on these assessments.

## 4,000 BABIES CAN'T BE WRONG

Over 4,000 mothers in Bogota have walked out the door of the maternity hospital with their premies snugly bound on their chests. The mothers kept their infants there continuously, twenty-four hours a day for a year, "wearing" them even as they slept, ate, worked, and cleaned house. (This, of course, may be difficult if not impossible for U.S. women!) Over the long term, Drs. Martínez and Rey, the originators of Kangaroo Care in Bogota, found that these home-kangarooed babies continued to grow exceptionally well. The infants who were cared for in this way:

- Were hospitalized less frequently than most premies are for recurring problems
- Had fewer respiratory difficulties
- Had fewer infections
- Continued to breastfeed
- Experienced no motor delays
- Looked healthy and vigorous
- Had nice round heads at one year of age

These findings have been confirmed by Dr. Figueroa de Leon, a physician at the Social Security Institute and Roosevelt Hospital, in Guatemala City, Guatemala. He has conducted one of the most comprehensive formalized evaluation of home-based Kangaroo Care to date. Dr. de Leon found that when this procedure is used at home for at least six months:

- Premies' weight gain was adequate, with some babies even gaining 5 to 10 grams more per day than premies not in home Kangaroo Care.

- Mothers were more likely to breastfeed exclusively (78 percent as compared to only 34 percent of non-Kangaroo Care mothers).
- Mothers breastfed much longer and consequently used less artificial formula.
- Mothers were more motivated to come back to the hospital for follow-up. (Some liked to return regularly to show off their babies because they were doing so well!)
- Mothers knew how to use hospital resources better.
- Premies required fewer nursing visits at home.

All in all, Dr. de Leon found many advantages and no adverse effects on growth and development when a premie is kangarooed at home. Home-based Kangaroo Care is clearly beneficial to you and your baby and is certainly worth a try.

## WHEN IS MY BABY READY FOR HOME KANGAROO CARE?

If your baby is well enough to go home, he's most likely gaining weight regularly, tolerating his feedings well, and having no significant breathing problems. With warmth, food, nurturing, and love—whether he weighs 1,800 grams (4 pounds) or 2,200 grams (nearly 5 pounds), whether he's 32 or 36 weeks—you can anticipate that he'll be physiologically stable and behaviorally responsive enough to tolerate less vigilant observation and have excellent chances to continue to grow and become healthy.

Under these circumstances, you can safely kangaroo your newborn at home. Rest assured that he'll be able to adapt to all of the normal shifting routines that go on in a home—the curious visitors, a sister coming home from preschool, the hubbub of early morning activity in your household.

Some premies are sent home with breathing monitors or oxygen tanks. They, too, can benefit from home Kangaroo Care. It's best, however, to obtain the discharge nurse's approval before beginning at home. You may need some additional instruction on how to manage the monitor or oxygen tank while kangarooing. You'll especially want to guard against dislodging the oxygen cannula. If your premie is dependent on this medical equipment, it may be easiest to continue kangarooing only while you're seated.

## HOW TO KANGAROO AT HOME

Kangaroo Care at home couldn't be easier. Just *wear your baby* as you carry out household chores. Films of Latin American Kangaroo Care mothers wearing their babies in a simple wrap or sling demonstrated that these women could do anything around the house including cooking, vacuuming, washing laundry, and washing the floors—activities that often involved stooping and bending over. The women even kept their babies in the kangaroo position when they went to bed at night, without rolling over on them.

How should you begin? First you need good hygiene. Wash your hands and have a shower. Second, simply diaper your infant, leaving his chest bare as it was in the hospital. Put him right up against your skin, holding him in place with a baby sling or pouch. (Snugli's "Legacy" sling and NoJo's "Original Baby Sling" are excellent choices. Both are available at Toys R Us stores.)

Don't wear a bra. The sling that will be supporting your baby will also shore up your breasts. Cover yourself with some loose-fitting clothing—an oversized blouse, smock, or robe will do just fine. Once you've gotten your infant set up, simply go about your daily business.

If you think you're catching a cold, it's best to ask your health care provider if you can continue Kangaroo Care while wearing a mask. Most moms are able to kangaroo using a mask even if they have the sniffles.

## HOW LONG SHOULD I KANGAROO AT HOME?

Usually from 40 to 52 weeks postconception, a baby's sleeping patterns will become stabilized. This is significant because adequate sleep is needed for brain maturation. And the regu-

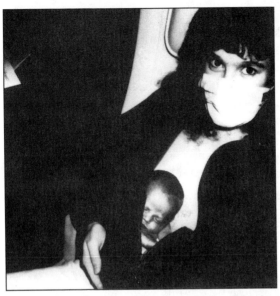

This mother is kangarooing in a mask to protect her child from her cold.

larity of sleep cycling is a marker of the establishment of circadian rhythm. (See Chapter 4, "Life in the Neonatal Intensive Care Unit.") Since Kangaroo Care may facilitate the development of prolonged periods of good sleep, I believe it's especially important for you to kangaroo your child at home until he is 52 weeks postconception.

Throughout this book, I've advocated kangarooing your premie at least an hour a day. The hospital routine and your schedule may not allow for more. But, in truth, I believe the more you hold your infant, the better. Researchers have gathered enough data to know that babies carried in slings are less fussy, better feeders, and better sleepers at 6 months than babies who are not carried. This should certainly pertain to Kangaroo Care babies as well. So, just when you think kangarooing might be coming to an end, it should be the beginning again—only this time at home.

And so I suggest kangarooing continuously for as long as possible and as frequently as possible during your infant's first 3 months of life (or until he reaches 52 weeks postconception).

The more the better. After all, Kangaroo Care enhances closeness between you and your infant!

As you get ready to leave the house, whenever you pull out an infant carrier or stroller, ask yourself, Could I be wearing my baby instead? The answer will most likely be, Yes. Of course, if you're taking your baby in a car, by law he must be secured in an infant seat. But once you get out, by love he should be on your chest. In fact, one of the easiest ways to use this loving procedure for several hours at a time is to kangaroo in bed.

## KANGAROOING IN BED

The South American mothers followed by Drs. Rey and Martínez have taken their babies to bed in Kangaroo Care. They kept their infants close by binding them onto their chests. If you're at work during the day and can't kangaroo your infant, then why not grab some time with him in bed?

If your infant is asleep, don't awaken him for Kangaroo

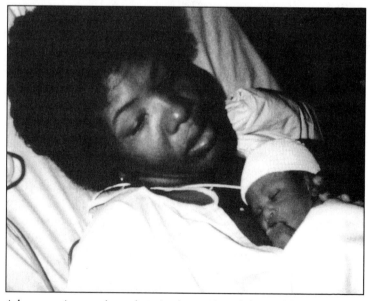

A kangarooing mother asleep in the semi-upright position.

Care. But if he is already up for a feeding, you can naturally move him into bedtime Kangaroo Care.

To try kangarooing in bed, be sure that you sleep in a semi-upright position, supported by two or three pillows. You'll want to make sure that your baby is upright to facilitate his breathing. And, when he goes to the breast during the night for sucking, you don't want him to regurgitate his feeding. The upright position helps the milk stay down. Eventually, you'll fall asleep and your baby will too. The good news is, you'll experience near-effortless nighttime feeding.

I don't want to mislead you, however. Sleeping semi-upright may be difficult to become accustomed to. You should know that it takes two to three days to develop good sleeping patterns and an awareness of where your baby is in bed with you. Rest assured that no mother has ever reported rolling over on her baby in the middle of the night.

You may worry that keeping your child in your bed will interfere with intimacy, but the fact is that premature babies usually sleep in their parents' rooms for the first few months of life anyway. Most fathers understand that the baby has been quite sick and are more than willing to go along with the new regime. Besides, they know it won't last forever.

## REGRESSION AND SIBLING RIVALRY

As Susan and Dr. Mitch Golant explain in their book *Getting Through to Your Kids* (Lowell House, 1991), when a new baby comes into the house, older siblings often respond by *regressing*. Regression means that a youngster reverts to childish behavior that he has already outgrown, such as bed-wetting, thumb sucking, helplessness, or tantrums.

Children perceive the birth of a sibling as a grave threat to their security. Your absence during the birth of the baby, the delay in bringing a premie home, and your frequent visits to the hospital have all increased the tension. In regressing, your youngster indirectly communicates to you that he is feeling stressed, frightened, or insecure. He asks for reassurance in the form of the nurturance that he sees you are providing the baby—especially a premie, who requires additional attention, and who is clearly enjoying the special closeness of kangarooing.

Can you help your older child get through this difficult period? Paradoxically, because of her vulnerable state, the more that you demand that your youngster "grow up," the less likely that she will heed you. You can help her overcome her regression by accepting her upset feelings and allowing her to act out the baby role more consciously. Allowing this acting out is an important way to validate your firstborn's emotions while removing the mystique of babyhood.

This means, for example, allowing your child to nurse at your breast, if she asks to and if it's not distasteful to you. She will find, of course, that your milk is quite bitter and may express surprise at the baby's apparent delight in drinking it. If your youngster is too old to nurse, you can offer her a bottle of formula to taste, or allow her to try out the crib. Let her lie skin-to-skin with you for a while, too, if she wants. And make sure that she gets one-to-one attention from her father, as well.

All that she may want is to be cuddled in the rocking chair as you sing an old lullaby. The more you allow her to act out her fantasy, the less powerful a hold it may have on her. In all likelihood, she'll be happy to return to her more grown-up life.

Sometimes young children have violent thoughts about their new sibling. Your older child may tell you to "take that sick baby back to the hospital," and make other hostile and upsetting remarks. As vulnerable as you are feeling, try not to overreact. Make it clear that no roughness is permitted around the baby, but acknowledge that big brothers and sisters often feel angry and scared about the changes in the family. You can use dolls, a punching bag, puppets, clay, drawing, or storytelling to help your youngster vent some of her feelings. If you are concerned about your older child's behavior, or if the situation doesn't improve, you may wish to consult your pediatrician for advice.

# EVERYONE JOINS IN

Mothers get so attached to the babies on their chest, they may have trouble relinquishing the infants to grandparents or other family members. But it's important for everyone in the family to feel that he or she is contributing to the baby's well-being. Close relatives have to become acquainted with the child, just as you do. More important, they also want to be able to help this child who has gotten off to a less than optimal start. Knowing that they're nurturing your infant enables them to feel that their help is of some consequence.

That's why all close family members may want to kangaroo your baby as long as they have no colds, infections, gastrointestinal upsets, or fevers and they wash their hands very well. Dr. de Leon of Guatemala has everyone in the family take over—fathers, grandparents, aunts and uncles, even siblings. But before you allow other family members to kangaroo your newborn, confirm the advisability of this practice with your child's health professional.

I have observed older sisters and brothers (from about the age of 7 years) kangarooing their premature siblings. They do it while sitting on the sofa, watching TV at night, or reading bedtime stories to the newborn. Walking around with the baby is difficult for them because they are unable to balance the infant's weight.

Your baby may start to suckle while being held by a family member, as he doesn't yet differentiate whether that individual's breast has milk. In that case, your relative should offer as a substitute a clean pacifier in your baby's mouth, just as the father may have done. (See Chapter 11, "Breastfeeding During Kangaroo Care.") As soon as your infant sucks on the pacifier, your family member should gently direct his mouth away from the breast.

Having these extra support people take over is also important for you, as it will give you some respite, allowing you a bit of time to get off to the shower or to run errands. For your own well-being, it's important for you to arrange time for yourself, too.

# WHAT TO DO IF YOU MUST GO BACK TO WORK

Most mothers of premies (or of full-term infants, for that matter) don't want to go right back to work. They feel that their babies are too fragile and vulnerable to be left with others. But the day of separation eventually comes, and it is fraught with uncertainty and concerns, especially because resources to care for premies are limited, hard to find, and difficult to evaluate.

When should you return to work? Ideally, it's wise to wait until your baby is at least 3 months older than your original full-term date because good day-night and sleep cycles are not usually set until then.

Separation from your baby is always difficult. If you've been kangarooing, it can be even more trying because you feel so attached to your infant. In fact, the decision to return to work can be agonizing because financial realities often don't coincide with emotional preferences.

Unfortunately, in most cases, you won't be able to take your baby to work with you. I eagerly await the day our society becomes more flexible and more tolerant of the need for babies and mothers to be together. But until that day, you'll rely on a sitter or child-care center. Should these caregivers kangaroo your infant? I'm not ready to advocate that they do. There's always a danger of infection. Child-care workers are exposed to many different children during the day, and it's not likely that they'll scrub down before holding your baby skin-to-skin. So begin kangarooing your infant as soon as practical once you get home from work. This is another instance where family members can also jump in and help out.

As you pick up your baby, you'll see how eager he is to be snuggled on your chest. He'll start nuzzling and gesturing as if to pull your clothing away to get that all-important skin-to-skin contact. Then, of course, he'll calm down as you place him in the secure, satisfying position that he seems to crave.

# WEANING YOUR INFANT AND YOURSELF

The research into Kangaroo Care is too young for us to have all the answers about its use at home. So, until results that suggest more stringent guidelines become available, use your own best judgment. If you don't feel like kangarooing from time to time, don't do it! You're entitled to time off, too.

When the daily routine of Kangaroo Care gets to be too much for you—your infant may become too hot, heavy, or hungry—then it may be time to wean yourselves from the practice. In order to do this slowly, dress your baby in a T-shirt and place him on the bed beside you. Let him lie slightly separated from your body at first. Move him away from you gradually, until he's about a pillow's width away. It may take two to three weeks of this physical distancing before your infant sleeps soundly without you.

Dr. William Sear's book *Nighttime Parenting* (La Leche League, 1985) is an excellent resource guide for the weaning and care of your premie during the night. It's available through the La Leche League and in many Toys R Us stores.

# EPILOGUE

# Kangaroo Care: Caring and Curing

In many parts of the world, when a premature infant is born at home, doctors and midwives immediately place him on his mother's chest, even prior to the cutting of the umbilical cord. This practice, common in France, Scandinavia, Africa, India, Central and South America, the Philippines, and Malaysia, is known as "early contact" but is, in reality, *immediate Kangaroo Care.*

Our society has grown distant from this humane and natural practice. Because premature babies can be quite ill at birth, we have developed technology-based strategies (such as artificial surfactants, ventilators, and warming trays) to take care of their many problems. We feel safe with these procedures and technologies, which have become increasingly efficient and effective in saving babies' lives.

We feel comfortable using medical standards that require us to take a premie directly to the NICU and hook him up to the available equipment and console ourselves that eventually, as he becomes stronger and healthier, his mother will have contact with him even when those medical standards may be compounding the stress the infant has to endure and may contribute to the very problems they are supposed to treat.

Yet it saddens me that our culture separates mothers and

babies in intensive care nurseries, especially when the lessons of 40,000 years of humankind have taught us that mothers seek contact with their infants and that children thrive when they achieve closeness with their parents. Now our job is to learn how to incorporate all of the phenomenal life-saving technological measures that we have come to depend on in the intensive care nursery with Mother Nature's design for natural care.

Research has already shown us that Kangaroo Care is a potent intervention, treatment, and form of contact. As we continue to investigate the subtle linkages between mother and baby that occur during Kangaroo Care, I'm convinced that we will find additional support for maintaining loving touch between mothers and their premies.

I have a dream that is neither grandiose nor impossible. My dream is that every premature baby 30 weeks gestation or more will be put on his mother's chest immediately after delivery and remain there so that his mother will become the intensive care bed for the duration of the premie's hospital stay. Smaller babies, too, can find comfort on their mothers' chests as soon as they are stabilized in the standard neonatal intensive care unit.

So much communication and symbiosis between mothers and babies occurs hormonally, chemically, electrically, and tactually! For this reason, I am sure that if we just give Kangaroo Care a chance, our premature infants will derive innumerable natural benefits, many of them as yet unknown. We won't be depending just on medicine. We'll also be depending on the intuitive, spontaneous, and mutual care-giving born of love that is our universal human gift.

# APPENDIX A

# Introducing Kangaroo Care to Your Hospital

If you've been told that you might experience a preterm birth, ask if your hospital offers Kangaroo Care. If not, you may want to discuss with your doctor how best to introduce it before you deliver. I have found that three key points must be communicated in order to convince a new institution to try this loving procedure.

*1. PUBLISHED RESEARCH*

The medical and nursing staff must have access to the full scope of research reports on Kangaroo Care in professional journals. The documentation of research is ongoing, since new studies emerge regularly. To simplify matters, there is one excellent article that reviews all the research studies through 1991. This article is written by Gene Cranston Anderson, Ph.D., and is entitled "Current Knowledge About Skin-to-Skin (Kangaroo) Care for Preterm Infants." It can be found in the September 1991 issue of the *Journal of Perinatology* (volume 11, number 3, pp. 216–26).

Another important source of information for all hospital staff is a very brief review article written by Andrew Whitelaw and entitled "Kangaroo Baby Care: Just a Nice Experience or an Important Advance for Preterm Infants?" In this article, which appeared in *Pediatrics* (1990, volume 85, pp. 604–5), Dr. Whitelaw encourages the use of Kangaroo Care for all babies in open-air cribs.

Ongoing research can be located through a computer search using the key words SKIN-TO-SKIN CONTACT or KAN-GAROO CARE. The staff at your hospital will have access to such an on-line medical database.

Gay Gale's forthcoming book entitled *Skin-to-Skin Holding: Handbook for NICU Caregivers* (Vort Publishers, Palo Alto, CA, 1993) spells out techniques for hospital staff using Kangaroo Care.

The following two articles are also useful:

Gene C. Anderson, E. A. Marks, and V. Walhlberg, "Kangaroo Care for Premature Infants," in the *American Journal of Nursing*, 1986, volume 86, pp. 807–9.

Gene C. Anderson, "Skin-to-Skin Kangaroo Care in Western Europe," in the *American Journal of Nursing*, 1989, volume 89, pp. 662–66.

All hospital libraries will have access to these journals.

It would also be helpful to let the neonatal intensive care unit staff know that the Maternal-Child branch of the World Health Organization supports the use and research of Kangaroo Care in many international settings. At this time, UNICEF is actively encouraging Kangaroo Care in Latin American and Caribbean hospitals and neonatal intensive care units. In 1988, UNICEF produced a 14-minute instructional video entitled *Mother Kangaroo—A Light of Hope* to encourage the use of Kangaroo Care. It's available in English or Spanish from:

UNICEF TV and Video Unit
H95, 3 U.N. Plaza
New York, NY 10017
(212) 326-7745

UNICEF published an English-language review of world-wide research on Kangaroo Care in Bogota, Colombia. It is entitled *First International Congress: The Kangaroo Care Program*, 1990.

In the United States, the National Institutes of Health, National Center for Nursing Research is supporting the advancement of Kangaroo Care by funding research studies of its benefits to premature infants and their families. Hospital staff can inquire at the National Institutes of Health in Bethesda, Maryland, for more information.

Articles on Kangaroo Care have appeared in newspapers and magazines. I've listed some of these articles chronologically.

Catherine Ione Sims, "Kangaroo Care," *Mothering*, Fall 1988.

"That Magic Touch," *Parents*, February 1989.

Peg Meier, "Kangaroo Care Adds Touch to High Tech," *St. Paul Star Tribune*, July 2, 1990.

D. Schulz, "Kangaroo Care," *Parents*, December 1990.

Nancy Stesin, "Hugs That Heal: Cuddling Skin-to-Skin," *Ladies' Home Journal*, January 1991.

Elizabeth Rosenthal, "Kangaroo's Pouch Inspires Care for Premature Babies," *The New York Times*, June 10, 1992, Living section.

## 2. KANGAROO CARE IN THE UNITED STATES

It is important for an intensive care unit to know where Kangaroo Care is practiced in the United States. Following is a partial list of hospitals at which Kangaroo Care is being practiced routinely at this time. If the staff at your hospital writes to the head nurse of a unit or the chief of neonatology, these professionals can summarize their experiences with Kangaroo Care.

## California
Doctor's Medical Center
Intensive Care Nursery
1441 Florida Avenue
Modesto, CA 95351
(209) 576-3737

Kaiser-Permanente Hospital
Nursing Department
280 W. MacArthur Boulevard
Oakland, CA 94611
(510) 596-7557

Children's Hospital of Oakland
Neonatal Intensive Care Unit
747 52nd Street
Oakland, CA 94609
(510) 428-3000 ext. 4956

Valley Presbyterian Hospital
Neonatal Intensive Care Unit
15107 Vanowen Street
Van Nuys, CA 81409
(818) 782-6600

## Colorado
Denver Children's Hospital
Neonatal Intensive Care Unit
1056 E. 19th Street
Denver, CO 80218
(303) 861-6857

## Florida
All Children's Hospital
Intensive Care Nursery
801 6th Street, South
St. Petersburg, FL 33731
(813) 898-7451

## Georgia
Emory University Hospital at Crawford-Long
Intermediate Nursery
550 Peachtree Street
Atlanta, GA 30365
(404) 686-2611

## Massachusetts
Brigham and Women's Hospital
Neonatal Intensive Care Unit
75 Francis Street
Boston, MA 02115
(617) 732-5500

## Minnesota
Children's Hospital of St. Paul
Neonatal Intensive Care Unit
345 N. Smith
St. Paul, MN 55102
(612) 220-6210

## Washington
Swedish Hospital
Special Care Nursery
747 Summit Avenue
Seattle, WA 98104
(206) 386-6000


*3. RESEARCH ON KANGAROO CARE IN THE
UNITED STATES*

The medical staff will want to know what Kangaroo Care research is currently being conducted in the United States. That will help them determine benefits of the procedure with patients, settings, and the types of medical problems and technology common in U.S. hospitals. (Research pertaining to problems in Colombia may not apply to your baby's situation or to your hospital.)

Research in Kangaroo Care is being conducted under the direction of those listed below at the following sites:

Susan M. Ludington-Hoe, C.N.M, Ph.D.
Associate Professor
UCLA School of Nursing
10833 Le Conte Ave.
Los Angeles, CA 90024-6919

Mercy Southwest Hospital
Annie Hollingsead, Acting Director of OB Services
400 Old River Road
Bakersfield, CA 93311

Francis Payne Bolton School of Nursing
Gene Cranston Anderson, RN, Ph.D., F.A.A.N.
Mellen Professor of Nursing
Case Western Reserve University
10900 Euclid Avenue
Cleveland, OH 44106-4904

Kadlec Medical Center
Joan Swinth, RNC, BSN
Neonatal Intensive Care Unit
888 Swift Boulevard
Richland, WA 99352

Please feel free to send a self-addressed stamped envelope for a list of the latest hospital sites using Kangaroo Care. By the same token, if Kangaroo Care is initiated in your hospital as a result of your efforts, please let me know. You may reach me at my U.C.L.A. School of Nursing office as follows:

Susan Ludington-Hoe, C.N.M., Ph.D.
U.C.L.A. School of Nursing
10833 Le Conte Avenue
Los Angeles, CA 90024-6919

# Current Research on When to Use Kangaroo Care

Dr. Gene Cranston Anderson has identified different time periods at which Kangaroo Care can begin. The research supporting the use of Kangaroo Care during each of these periods is described below. This material will provide a brief summary of all the latest research for hospital staff.

## BIRTH KANGAROO CARE

To date, there are no published scientific reports analyzing the benefits of the immediate placement of the premature baby against his mother's chest prior to the cord being cut and the infant's condition being medically assessed.

But hospitals around the world are routinely practicing birth Kangaroo Care and have had no problems with it in infants who are 34 to 36 weeks gestational age and have 5-minute APGARs of 6 or more. These hospitals are in Sweden, Germany, Denmark, Mexico, and Guatemala. Medical personnel at several of these institutions have assured me that the babies do well in immediate Kangaroo Care, as long as they meet the above criteria.

Several of these hospitals are now gathering specific clinical data about how the babies adapt to birth Kangaroo Care so that others might be able to try it, too.

## VERY EARLY KANGAROO CARE

Pioneering efforts have been made in establishing the scientific value of very early Kangaroo Care, which begins within the first 30 minutes of life. Because it is customary practice in the United States for a premature infant to be handed over to a neonatal team immediately to assess his specific needs and problems, the earliest that Kangaroo Care has been practiced is after health professionals assess the infant's condition, dry him off, and see how he adapts to the first 5 to 10 minutes of extrauterine life.

It is common in France, Denmark, and Sweden for babies to be handed right back to their mothers for Kangaroo Care within five minutes of birth even if the infants are 27 or 28 weeks gestation. (These are tiny babies!)

The earliest I have been able to place a baby in Kangaroo Care in our studies is at 12 minutes after birth. This occurred during my research at the Hospital Universitario del Valle in Cali, Colombia with Dr. Gene Cranston Anderson. We needed those minutes to dry the infant, assess his breathing and heart rate, and attach all of our monitoring electrodes. We returned the baby to his mother as she reclined on the delivery table and we completed her delivery.

Kangaroo Care was accompanied by great benefit to the baby: Immediately we saw him warming up, even though he was naked (but covered by the standard hospital receiving blanket folded in fourths). The infant relaxed so well that soon his breathing became quite regular and unlabored. His oxygen saturation levels started to climb immediately and quickly reached the normal range.

We continued this study with six babies and perfected our routines regarding how to care for mother and baby in research conditions.

Experience with very early Kangaroo Care led to two further investigations. First, we engaged in a very sophisticated comparison study in which one group of babies began Kangaroo Care in the delivery room whereas the control group received routine open-air crib care. The results are showing that healthy premature babies can be safely kangarooed during the first six hours of life.

In the second study, Dr. Anderson returned to the University of Florida and secured the involvement of Brigitte Syfrette, a nurse-midwife who was in graduate school. They decided to try Kangaroo Care starting in the delivery room with babies who are born 4 to 6 weeks early. They asked the mothers to continue to hold their babies until the mothers were to be discharged, 24 hours after delivery. The mothers carried their babies in pouches as they walked around the postpartum unit. They even slept with their infants on their chests.

When Dr. Anderson saw how well these babies were doing, she brought the infants into the hospital's clinical research center. There they stayed with their mothers for another day or two for further study.

As a result of this research, we know that the babies stayed very warm as long as they remained skin-to-skin with their mothers. They became competent breastfeeders within 24 hours, and after only a few days they began to gain weight. In fact, the babies experiencing Kangaroo Care needed hospitalization for just 3.7 days. In contrast, premies who went directly to the intensive care unit (without Kangaroo Care) remained in the hospital for 10 days.

This pilot study will be used to guide a comparison study in the United States using many more babies, duplicating the study conducted on very early Kangaroo Care in Florida.

## EARLY KANGAROO CARE

Early Kangaroo Care begins as soon as the baby is stabilized after birth or within the first 24 hours of life. Babies on ventilators are included in this group.

To date, three studies have assessed the effects of early Kangaroo Care. Dr. Moeller-Jensen and his associates at the

Soenderborg Hospital in Soenderborg, Denmark, placed infants under 1,500 grams in Kangaroo Care within the first day of life. He noted that the procedure had an immediate positive impact on the infants' temperature, pulse, and respiration.

Allowing mothers to hold and carry their premies in the ward, Dr. Moeller-Jensen soon learned that the babies became quite warm during Kangaroo Care and require less clothing. He found that, after a few days of being carried by the mothers, these babies were more awake, sought their mothers' faces, and were eager to suck.

Dr. Richard de Leeuw at the Academic Medical Center, University of Amsterdam, the Netherlands, has researched Kangaroo Care extensively with over one hundred babies. He allows any relatively stabilized newborn admitted to the NICU to start Kangaroo Care with a ventilator in place.

Mothers and fathers come into the Academic Medical Center and hold their babies for as long and as often as they want. Dr. de Leeuw has found that parents usually stay a minimum of 30 minutes. He has had the same wonderful results that we have: The infants' skin temperatures go up and their breathing patterns normalize while they're being held. And perhaps most important, he found that the infection rate is no greater for babies held in Kangaroo Care than for babies who are not.

As a result of his research, Dr. de Leeuw has concluded that Kangaroo Care is a safe method even for tiny, nonstabilized babies. Their medical condition does not deteriorate. He has never needed to stop Kangaroo Care because of a clinical problem.

## INTERMEDIATE KANGAROO CARE

Intermediate Kangaroo Care begins after 7 days of hospitalization when infants are stabilized and in incubators. It begins after the infant is taken off the ventilator. A great deal of research has been carried out on these premies in Germany, Finland, England, and the United States.

Again, the findings are consistent: Babies experience improvement in oxygenation, breathing patterns, and warmth while in Kangaroo Care. (Mothers warm babies better than incubators; breathing patterns become almost perfectly normal during Kangaroo Care.)

All the parents like the procedure. Breastfeeding is fostered because mothers produce more milk; mothers who have engaged in Kangaroo Care tend to breastfeed for longer periods. In one study, babies in intermediate Kangaroo Care were discharged an average of 7 days earlier than those who had not experienced the procedure, and they cried significantly less at 6 months of age.

Dr. Eberhardt Schmidt at the University of Dusseldorf, Germany, found that mothers using Kangaroo Care form stronger bonds with their babies. He allowed mothers in his study to start holding their infants as soon as they graduated to incubators. His primary focus was feeding behavior and infection. Dr. Schmidt found that 50 percent of the Kangaroo Care mothers were breastfeeding while none of the controls were. Kangaroo Care mothers had more milk production than the other mothers, resulting in better growth for their infants, and there was no increase in the rate of infection over the control group.

At Kadlec Medical Center in Richland, Washington, I wanted to use Kangaroo Care with babies who still needed incubators for temperature control. I reasoned that if Kangaroo Care helped older babies retain body warmth, it should help younger ones, too.

We started by watching the babies for three hours in their incubators. Then, we had the mothers hold the babies for three hours. Finally, we watched the premies for another three hours after they were returned to their incubators. We were concerned about the babies' ability to maintain their temperature and remain stable in light of all the stimulation they would be getting on their mothers' chests: listening to the heartbeat and voice, being rhythmically moved, touched, and contained.

In a pilot study involving four Kangaroo Care babies, we found a good deal of apnea and periodic breathing in the pre–Kangaroo Care period. During Kangaroo Care, apnea reduced dramatically. It was entirely eliminated in three babies. The fourth still experienced some breathing difficulties, but the apnea occurred much less frequently in Kangaroo Care than in the incubator.

When trying to figure out why this baby was experiencing apnea, we noticed that he was so relaxed in Kangaroo Care, he literally scrunched down: His body compressed as he tucked himself, flexed in, and became tension free. We noted that whenever he became so completely relaxed, he would have an apnea attack. It occurred to us that the degree of relaxation might have contributed to a form of apnea called *obstructive apnea*, in which the air flow into the lungs is impeded.

None of the previous studies had identified whether apneas during Kangaroo Care were obstructive or were caused by immaturity of the brain (a form called *central apnea*). We decided that we had better find out, especially if we wanted to be sure that Kangaroo Care was safe for incubator babies. So we began a new study. To date, we have collected data on 17 Kangaroo Care and 15 control babies. We have seen a fourfold decrease in central apnea during Kangaroo Care and no increase in obstructive apnea in infants weighing 2,000 grams or more.

We learned that if a baby is limp, flaccid, and weak, he may be unable to keep his chest expanded during Kangaroo Care in an upright position. Mothers of these small babies need to recline more than sit up. Rather than placing these infants in an upright position, we angle them so that they're resting on one breast or the other. If the infant should bend his head forward as he falls asleep, we reposition his head, straightening it to make sure his airway stays open. In addition, many of these smaller babies should be watched closely in the first half hour after feeding to avoid gastro-esophageal reflux.

We are now letting our mothers hold the babies for five consecutive days in Kangaroo Care to see if the beneficial effects we get on the first day continue.

# LATE KANGAROO CARE

Late Kangaroo Care begins when a baby is able to breathe room air and is in an open-air crib. Kangaroo Care boasts many benefits at this stage: Babies become competent breastfeeders, sleep well, cry little, start to become alert, and interact with their parents. They show good growth patterns. These are the babies most readily available for Kangaroo Care, and they comprise the largest proportion of premie babies studied.

My team and I carried out our first study in 1988, with twelve open-air crib babies (they were getting ready for discharge) at the Hollywood Presbyterian Hospital in Los Angeles. Usually, we've removed these babies' monitors because we believe they're relatively stable. For the purposes of the research study, however, we reattached the wires. We watched the babies for three hours before Kangaroo Care, gave them to the mothers for three hours of Kangaroo Care, and then watched them again for three hours after Kangaroo Care.

We were surprised to see how many of these babies were still experiencing abnormal breathing patterns in the three hours before and after Kangaroo Care—this, just prior to discharge! When the neonatologist saw the data, he initiated a practice of recording the babies' breathing patterns before they go home. The recording is called a "pneumogram." Many hospitals will obtain a 12-hour pneumogram during the night to determine if the baby needs to go home with an apnea monitor.

But during Kangaroo Care, breathing patterns were normal. We found neither apnea nor periodic breathing with babies in open-air cribs.

These results were so encouraging that we decided to move into a randomized control clinical trial, a sophisticated design that enables us to select babies and assign them to receive the treatment (Kangaroo Care) or not (control). We compare the data and evaluate what changes were due to the Kangaroo Care, which gives us some understanding of cause and effect.

This randomized control trial was conducted with 13 Kangaroo Care babies and 11 control babies at Kadlec Medical

Center in Richland, Washington. It revealed the same results: During Kangaroo Care babies got warm and enjoyed significant reductions in apnea and periodic breathing. They doubled the amount of time spent in sleep and dramatically reduced the time spent in purposeless activity.

Based on the results with the randomized control trial of one day of Kangaroo Care with babies in open-air cribs, the National Institutes of Health, National Center for Nursing Research, the federal agency that supports health-related research, granted me funds to continue work with incubator babies to determine if the benefits we saw continued for five days. In this study, which is in progress at Little Company of Mary Hospital, in Torrance, California, we're also looking at feeding behaviors, at alleviation of infant and maternal stress, and at discharge dates and length of hospitalization.

Research on Kangaroo Care is proceeding, even if at times the progress seems slow. When any new treatment is tested, the research program must be expanded in a cautious, deliberate, and logical way, so the safety of the treatment can be determined. As you have read, there are many different types of premies, different Kangaroo Care starting times, and different amounts of Kangaroo Care to be evaluated. All of these evaluations require time. Yet, similar benefits have been shown by so many studies that now is the time to start using this treatment with all open-air crib premies.

# APPENDIX C

# Metric Conversions

30 grams = 1 ounce
450 grams = 1 pound
1° centigrade = 5–9° Fahrenheit
37° centigrade = 98.6° Fahrenheit
38° centigrade = 100.4° Fahrenheit

# Glossary

**Apnea.** Periods in which the premie "forgets" to breathe.

**Artificial surfactants.** Medications that help the premie's lungs become more elastic.

**Betamethasone.** A medication that helps the infant's lungs mature.

**Blow-by oxygen.** An oxygen-emitting tube placed by the infant's nose to supplement oxygen supply.

**Bradycardia.** Slow heartbeat, under 120 beats per minute.

**Bradypnea.** Slow breathing rate. Respiratory rate drops below 30 breaths per minute.

**Cannula.** A small tube with prongs that delivers oxygen into the infant's nose without adding either pressure or volume.

**Central apnea.** Cessation of breathing caused by the brain.

**Continuous positive airway pressure (CPAP).** A setting on the ventilator machine that maintains a small amount of constant pressure to keep the airway open.

**Dexamethasone.** A medication that promotes lung maturity.

**Flexion.** The fetal position, with arms bent at the elbows and legs bent at the knees.

**Full-term baby.** Any baby born between 38 and 42 weeks gestation.

**Gastroesophageal reflux babies.** Premies with immature muscle tone in the stomach and esophagus who spit up frequently.

**Gavage feeding.** Introducing liquid food into the stomach by placing a tube down the infant's throat.

**Gestational age.** The number of weeks in the womb. Full-term pregnancy is 40 weeks long.

**Grunting respirations.** An early sign of respiratory distress. Babies emit these sounds as they instinctively try to prevent their lungs from collapsing by retaining some air within the passageway.

**Incubator.** An enclosed warming unit, usually made of clear plastic.

**Intraventricular hemorrhage.** Bleeding into the brain as a result of blood pressure changes within the brain.

**Intubation.** Placing a tube down the infant's throat into the lungs to insure the infant's lungs receive adequate oxygen.

**Jaundice.** Medical condition in which old red blood cells are not broken down by the infant's immature liver, causing them to collect under the skin and giving the skin a yellow tint. Jaundice is treated with lights that break down the blood cells.

**Latency to respond.** Premie takes time to process environmental input and change behavior.

**Medical touch.** Any touch related to therapy.

**Minimal handling baby.** A baby who can't tolerate frequent medical touching. Staff should consolidate treatments.

**Neonatologist.** A physician who specializes in the problems of newborn infants.

**Neutral thermal zone.** The temperature range at which a baby has minimal oxygen needs.

**Nippling baby.** An infant who is able to take nutrition by sucking on a bottle or a mother's breast.

**NPO.** Medical jargon which stands for nothing (no food or medication) by mouth.

**Obstructive apnea.** Breathing ceases because airflow to the lungs is impeded.

**Oxygen saturation (also $SaO_2$ or $O_2Sat$).** How much

oxygen the blood is carrying. Normal rates are 88 to 100 percent saturation.

**Oxytocin.** The hormone critical to the milk ejection reflex. It triggers the release of milk by causing the muscle cells surrounding the milk sacs to contract, and it also causes the muscles of the uterus to contract.

**Parenteral nutrition.** Nutritional fluid introduced directly into the blood.

**Percutaneous line.** An intravenous tube threaded through a vein in the arm to the heart by which nutrition is provided to the infant.

**Periodic breathing.** A situation in which there are at least three episodes of apnea alternating with deep catch-up breaths.

**Postconceptional age.** Weeks in the womb plus weeks out of the womb.

**Premature baby** ( also **preterm** or **premie**). Any baby born before 38 weeks gestation.

**Premie nipple.** A special bottle nipple that makes it easier for the milk to flow and prevents flooding of the mouth during feeding.

**Pulse oxymeter.** A sensor that measures the blood's oxygen saturation.

**Radiant warmer.** An open, flat bed that has a warming unit placed directly above the infant. Sicker premies are placed in radiant warmers for easy access.

**Random startle.** A reflex in which the baby kicks out his legs and spreads his arms wide, bringing them back into midline with tremors. (Also known as the *Moro reflex.*)

**Servo-control.** A small, flat disc that communicates an infant's body temperature to the warming unit of the radiant warmer or incubator so the warmer keeps the baby at the proper temperature.

**Social touch.** Soothing, calming, and affectionate touch.

**Tachycardia.** Rapid heartbeat of 160 or more beats per minute.

**Tachypnea.** Rapid breathing rate (can be 60 breaths per minute or more during crying).

**Theophylline.** A medication that regulates breathing.

**Thermoregulatory system.** The hypothalamus, blood vessels, skin, and sweat glands, which together help regulate an individual's temperature.

**Thermoregulatory behaviors.** The baby's stretching out of an arm or leg away from the body in order to cool down.

**Total parenteral feeding.** All nutrients are coming in through the infant's blood vessels. (Also called *TPN*.)

**Transcutaneous** (through the skin) **pressure of oxygen** **(TCPO$_2$).** A measure of the pressure of oxygen traveling in the blood cells right under the skin using a sensor.

**Umbilical artery catheter.** A small tube inserted into the umbilicus that enables care-givers to measure the internal blood pressure, blood flow, and blood oxygen levels and to get blood samples without having to repeatedly stick the infant. (Also called *U-line* or *UAC*.)

**Vasopressor.** A general term for medication that regulates blood pressure.

**Ventilator.** Machine that helps the infant breathe (also known as a *respirator*).

# References

Acolet, D., K. Sleath, and A. Whitelaw. 1989. Oxygenation, heart rate, and temperature in very low birth weight infants during skin-to-skin contact with their mothers. *Acta Paediatrica Scandinavica* 78, pp. 189–93.

Affonso D., E. Bosque, V. Wahlberg, and J. Brady. Reconciliation and healing for mothers through skin-to-skin contact provided in an American tertiary level intensive care nursery. *Neonatal Network,* April 1993, Vol. 12, No. 3, pp. 25–32.

Affonso, D., V. Wahlberg, and B. Persson. 1989. Exploration of mother's reactions to the Kangaroo method of prematurity care. *Neonatal Network* 7 (6), pp. 43–51.

Als, H. 1986. A synactive model of neonatal behavioral organization: Framework for the assessment of neurobehavioral development in the premature infant and for support of infants and parents in the neonatal intensive care environment. *Physical and Occupational Therapy in Pediatrics* 6 (3/4), pp. 3–37.

Anand, K.J.S., and P.R. Hickey. 1987. Pain and its effects in the human neonate and fetus. *New England Journal of Medicine* 317, pp. 1321–29.

Anderson, G.C. 1975. A preliminary report: Severe respiratory distress in transitional newborn lambs with recovery following nonnutritive sucking. *Journal Nurse Midwifery,* Summer, pp. 20–28.

Anderson, G.C. 1986. Pacifiers: The positive side. *American Journal of Maternal-Child Nursing,* 11, pp. 122–24.

Anderson, G.C. 1988. Crying, foramen ovale shunting, and cerebral volume. *Pediatrics 113,* pp. 411–12.

Anderson, G.C. 1989. Skin-to-skin: Kangaroo Care in Western Europe. *American Journal of Nursing* 89, pp. 662–66.

Anderson, G.C. 1991. Current knowledge about skin-to-skin (Kangaroo) care for preterm infants. *Journal of Perinatology,* 11, pp. 216–26.

Anderson, G.C., A.K. Burroughs, and C.P. Measel, 1983. Nonnutritive sucking opportunities: A safe and effective treatment for preterm neonates. In T. Field and A. Sostek, eds., *Infants Born At Risk,* Vol. 8, No. 5, N.Y.: Grune and Stratton, pp. 129–46.

Anderson, G.C., E.A. Marks, and V. Wahlberg. 1986. Kangaroo care for premature infants. *American Journal of Nursing,* 86, pp. 807–9.

Apostolakis, E.M. 1982. Visual Preferences of preterm and term infants. *California Journal of Perinatology,* Vol. 2, pp. 47–53.

Argote, L.A., H. Rey, S.M. Ludington-Hoe, G. Medallin, E. Casro, and G.C. Anderson. 1991. Dificultad respiratorio transitoria y contacto piel a piel temprano como manejo. *Proceedings of the 17th Colombian Pediatric Congress,* Bogota, Colombia, p. 532.

Armstrong, H.C. 1987. Breastfeeding low birth weight babies: Advances in Kenya. *Journal of Human Lactation* 3(2), pp. 34–37.

Avery, G.B., and P. Glass. 1986. Light and Retinopathy of prematurity: What is prudent for 1986? *Pediatrics* 78, pp. 519–20.

Bellefeuille-Reid, D., and S. Jakubec. 1989. Adaptive Positioning Intervention for premature infants: Issues for paediatric occupational therapy practice. *British Journal of Occupational Therapy,* 52(3), pp. 93–96.

Bernbaum, J.C. 1982. Increased oxygenation with nonnutritive sucking during gavage feedings in premature infants. *Pediatric Research* 16(4), Abstract 1199, p. 278A.

Bernbaum, J.C. 1983. Nonnutritive sucking during gavage feeding: Enhances growth and maturation of premature infants. *Pediatrics* 71, pp. 41–45.

Blackburn, S.T., and K.E. Barnard. 1985. Analysis of caregiving events relating to preterm infants in the special care unit. *Infant Stress Under Intensive Care.* Baltimore: University Park Press. pp. 113–30.

Blackburn, S. 1993. The use of orally directed behaviors by VLBW infants. *Neonatal Network* 12(2), p. 61.

Blackburn, S., and D. Patteson. 1991. Effects of cycled light on activity state and cardiorespiratory function in preterm infants. *J. Perinatal Neonatal Nursing,* Vol. 4, pp. 47–54.

Bosque, E.M., J. P. Brady, D.D. Affonso, and V. Wahlberg. 1988. Continuous physiologic measures of kangaroo versus incubator care in a tertiary level nursery. *Pediatric Research* 23 (4, part 2), Abstract 1204, p. 402A.

Bradley, R.M., and C.M. Mistretta. 1975. Fetal sensory receptors. *Psychological Review* 55, pp. 352–82.

Canestrini, S. 1913. On the sensory life of the newborn according to physiological experiments. *Santgebiete Neurological Psychiatrie* 5, pp. 1–104.

Catlett, A.T., and D. Holditch-Davis. 1990. Environmental stimulation of the acutely ill premature infant: Physiological effects and nursing implications. *Neonatal Network* 8, pp. 19–26.

Chaze, B.A., and S.M. Ludington-Hoe, 1984. Sensory stimulation in the NICU. *American Journal of Nursing* 84(1), pp. 68–71.

Cole, J.G., and P.A. Frappier. 1985. Infant stimulation reassessed: A new approach for providing care for the preterm infant. *Journal of Obstetric Gynecologic, and Neonatal Nursing* (November/December), pp. 471–77.

Collins, S.K., and K. Kuck. 1991. Music Therapy in the neonatal intensive care unit. *Neonatal Network* 9(6), pp. 23–26.

Collins, S. 1993. Baby Stephanie: A case study in compassionate care. *Neonatal Intensive Care,* March/April 1993, pp. 47–49.

Colonna, F., G. Uxa, A.M. de Graca, and U. de Wonderweld, 1990. The "Kangaroo-Mother" method: Evaluation of an alternative for the care of low birth weight newborns in developing countries. *International Journal of Gynecology and Obstetrics* 31, pp. 335–39.

De Casper, A.J., and A.D. Sigafoos. 1980. Of human bonding: Newborns prefer mother's voice. *Science* (June), pp. 51–53.

De Casper, A.J., and A.D. Sigafoos. 1983. The intrauterine heartbeat as a potent reinforcer for newborns. *Infant Behavior and Development* 6, pp. 19–25.

De Leeuw, R. 1986. The Kangaroo method. *Vraagbak: A Quarterly for Development Workers* 14(4), pp. 50–58.

De Leeuw, R. 1988. The Kangaroo-method in the care of preterm infants. Videotape and paper presented at the Eleventh European Congress of Perinatal Medicine, April 1988, Rome.

De Leeuw, R., E.M. Colin, E.A. Dunnebier, and M. Mirmiran. 1991. Physiological effects of kangaroo care in very small preterm infants. *Biology of the Neonate* 59, pp. 149–55.

de Leon, F. "The Kangaroo Care Method: Application and Use." Presentation at International Well Start, 8/20/92, San Diego.

Dowd, J.M., and E.Z. Tronick. 1986. Temporal coordination of arm movements in early infancy: Do infants move in synchrony with adult speech? *Child Development* 57, pp. 762–76.

Duxbury, J.L., et al. 1984. Caregiver disruptions and sleep of high risk infants. *Heart and Lung* 13, pp. 141–47.

Elliman, A.M., E.M. Bryan, A.D. Elliman, and D. Starte. 1986. Narrow heads of preterm infants: Do they matter? *Developmental Medicine and Child Neurology* 28, pp. 745–48.

Gabriel, M., B. Grote, and M. Jonas. 1981. Sleep-wake pattern in preterm infants under two different care schedules during four day polygraphic recording, *Neuropediatrics* 12, pp. 366–73.

Gale, G. 1993. *Skin-to-Skin Holding: Handbook for NICU Caregivers.* Palo Alto: Vort Publishers.

Gale, G., L. Branck, and C. Lund. Skin-to-skin holding of intubated premature infants. *Neonatal Network,* Vol. 12.

Gardner, S.L., J.P. O'Donnel, and L.E. Weisman, 1989. Breastfeeding the sick neonate. In Merenstein, G.B., and S.L. Gardner, eds., *Handbook of Neonatal Intensive Care.* St. Louis: C.V. Mosby. pp. 238–60.

Glass, P., G.B. Avery, and K.N. Subramanian. 1985. Effect of bright light in the hospital nursery on the incidence of retinopathy of prematurity. *New England Journal of Medicine* 313, pp. 401–4.

Goldberg, C., et al. 1983. Head positioning and intracranial pressures. *Critical Care Medicine* 11(6), pp. 428–30.

Gorski, P.A. 1991. Developmental Intervention during neonatal hospitalization. *Pediatrics Clinics of North America* 38(6), pp. 1469–79.

Gorski, P.A. 1991. Behavioral assessment of the newborn. In Taeusch, H., R. Ballard, and M. Avery, (eds.) *Diseases of the Newborn,* 6th ed. Philadelphia: W.B. Saunders. pp. 320–21.

Gorski, P.A., T.B. Brazelton, et al. 1979. Stages of behavioral organization in the high risk neonate: Theoretical and clinical considerations. *Seminars in Perinatology* 3(1), pp. 61–72.

Gorski, P.A., W.T. Hole, C.H. Leonard, and J.A. Martin. 1983. Direct computer recording of premature infants and nursery care: Distress following two interventions. *Pediatrics* 72, pp. 198–202.

Gottfried, A.W. 1985. Environment of newborn infants in special care units. In Gottfried, A.W., and J.L. Gaiter, eds., *Infant Stress Under Intensive Care.* Baltimore: University Park Press.

Hargboel, A. 1987. Luna—A child who has tried the Kangaroo Method. *Foraldre og Fodsel,* No. 1.

Heimler, R., J. Langlois, D.J. Hodel, L.D. Nelin, and P. Sasidharan. 1992. Effects of positioning on the breathing pattern of preterm infants. *Archives of Diseases in Childhood* 67, pp. 312–14.

Helders, P. 1989. The effects of a sensory stimulation/range-finding program on the development of very low birthweight infants. Ph.D. Dissertation, College van Dekanen, Nederlands.

Hemingway, M. and S. Oliver. 1991. Waterbed therapy and cranial molding of the sick preterm infant. *Neonatal Network* 10, pp. 32–35.

Hosseini, R.B., M.S. Hashemi, and S.M. Ludington-Hoe. 1992. Preterm infants and fathers: Physiologic and behavioral effects of skin-to-skin contact. *Ursus Medicus* 2, pp. 47–55.

Kellman, N. 1982. Noise in the intensive care nursery. *Neonatal Network* 2, pp. 8–17.

Koniak, D., S.M. Ludington-Hoe, B. Chaze, and S. Sachs. 1985. The impact of preterm birth on maternal perception of the neonate. *Journal of Perinatology* 5(3), pp. 29–35.

Korones, S. 1976. Disturbance and infant's rest. In Moore, T., ed., *Iatrogenic Problems in the NICU: Report of the 69th Ross Conference of Pediatric Research.* Columbus: Ross Labs. pp. 74–97.

Lamb, P. 1982. Early contact and maternal-infant bonding: One decade later. *Pediatrics* 70, pp. 763–68.

Langer, V.S. 1990. Minimal handling protocol for the intensive care nursery. *Neonatal Network* 9(3), pp. 23–27.

Leonard, J.E. 1993. Music Therapy: Fertile ground for application of research in practice. *Neonatal Network* 12(2), pp. 47–48.

Levene, S., and S.A. McKenzie. 1990. Transcutaneous oxygen saturation in sleeping infants: Prone and supine. *Archives of Diseases in Childhood* 65, pp. 524–26.

Long, J.G., J.F. Lucey, and A.G.S. Philip. 1980. Noise and hypoxemia in the intensive care nursery. *Pediatrics* 65, pp. 143–45.

Lucey, J.F. 1977. Is intensive care becoming too intensive? *Pediatric Neonatology Supplement* 59, pp. 1064–65.

Lucey, J.F. 1984. The sleeping, dreaming fetus meets the intensive care nursery. In *The Many Facets of Touch,* Johnson and Johnson Roundtable No. 10, p. 79.

Ludington-Hoe, S.M. 1983. What can newborns really see? *American Journal of Nursing* 83, pp. 1286–89.

————. 1987. Sensory enrichment with competent newborns. *Pediatric Nursing Forum* 2(2), pp. 3–13.

————. 1990. Energy conservation during Kangaroo Care. *Heart and Lung: Journal of Critical Care* 19, pp. 445–51.

————. 1992. Kangaroo care's effects on crying and agitation in preterm infants. *Proceedings of the "Challenge of Neonatal and Pediatric Nursing: Integrating Research into the Art of and Science of Clinical Practice."* Children's Hospitals of Southern California, pp. 106–7.

Ludington-Hoe, S.M., and G.C. Anderson. 1991. Preliminary results of very early kangaroo care for preterm infants. Paper presented at 8th National Meeting of the Nurse's Association of the American College of Obstetricians and Gynecologists, June 10, 1991, Orlando.

Ludington-Hoe, S.M., G.C. Anderson, and A. Hadeed. 1990. Maternal-neonatal thermal synchrony during skin-to-skin contact. Paper presented at International Congress of Infant Studies, April 9, 1990, Montreal.

Ludington-Hoe, S.M., G.C. Anderson, H. Rey, and L.A. Argote. 1992. Transitional physiology and state behavior of Colombian preterm infants in skin-to-skin (kangaroo) care and open-air cribs beginning in the delivery room. *Infant Behavior and Development* 15, p. 537 (abstract).

Ludington-Hoe, S.M., G.C. Anderson, S. Simpson, A. Hollingshead, L.A. Argote, and H. Rey. Skin-to-skin contact beginning in the delivery room for Colombian mothers and their preterm infants. For publication. *Journal of Human Lactation.*

Ludington-Hoe, S.M. and A.J. Hadeed. 1992. Kangaroo Care: Fourfold reduction in apnea. Paper presented at Southwestern Pediatric Society Annual Spring Meeting, May 8, 1992, Ojai, California.

Ludington-Hoe, S.M., A. Hadeed, and G.C. Anderson. 1991. Physiologic responses to skin-to-skin contact in hospitalized premature infants. *Journal of Perinatology* 11, pp. 19–24.

————. 1993. State regulation in premature infants during skin-to-skin contact with their mothers. Manuscript submitted for publication.

————. 1993. Synchrony in maternal and premature infant temperature during skin-to-skin contact. Manuscript submitted for publication.

Ludington-Hoe, S.M. and F. Hashemi. 1991. Temporal relationship between kangaroo care and crying. Paper presented at International Sigma Theta Tau Meeting, November 12, 1991, Tampa.

Ludington-Hoe, S.M., B. Hosseini, M.S. Hashemi, L.A. Argote, G. Medellin, and H. Rey. 1992. Selected physiologic measures and behavior during paternal skin contact with Colombian preterm infants. *Journal Developmental Physiology* 18, pp. 223–32.

Ludington-Hoe, S.M., C. Thompson, and J. Swinth. 1992. Efficacy of Kangaroo care with preterm infants in open-air cribs. *Neonatal Network* 11(6), p. 101.

————. 1994. Research program in kangaroo care: Collaboration, results, and practice implications. *Neonatal Network.*

Mann, N.P., R. Haddow, L. Stokes, S. Goodley, and N. Ruttern. 1986. Effect of night and day on preterm infants in a newborn nursery: Randomized trial. *British Medical Journal,* Vol. 293, pp. 1265–67.

McCain, N.P. 1992. Facilitating inactive awake states in preterm infants: A study of three interventions—nonnutritive sucking and rocking and stroking. *Nursing Research* 41(3), pp. 157–60.

Measel, C.P., and G.C. Anderson. 1979. Nonnutritive sucking during tube feedings: Effect on clinical course in premature infants. *Journal of Obstetrics, Gynecologic, and Neonatal Nursing,* 8, September/October, pp. 265–72.

Meier, P. 1980. A program to support breastfeeding in the high-risk nursery. *Perinatology/Neonatology* 5, p. 43.

Mellor, David H. and A.R. Fielder. 1980. Dissociated visual development: Electrodiagnostic studies in infants who are slow to see. *Developmental Medicine and Child Neurology* 22, pp. 327–35.

Miles, M.S. and M.C. Carter. 1983. Assessing parental stress in intensive care units. *Maternal Child Nursing* 8, pp. 354–59.

Miller, C.L., M.F. O'Callaghan, T.L. Whitman, and R. White. 1993. The effects of the NICU environment on infant behavior and development. Paper presented at the 60th Annual Society for Research in Child Development Conference, New Orleans, LA, March.

Miranda, S.B. 1970. Visual abilities and pattern preferences of preterm and fullterm infants. *Developmental Medicine and Child Neurology,* 10, pp. 189–205.

Mitchell, S.A. 1984. Noise pollution in the neonatal intensive care nursery. *Seminars in Hearing* 5(1), pp. 17–24.

Moeller-Jensen, H., K. Hjort-Gregersen, M. Matthiessen, H. Vestergard, and B.H. Jepson. 1987. The Kangaroo Method used in practice at the Hospital of Soenderborg, Denmark. English translation from Danish journal *Sygeplejersken (The Nurse)* by Larsen, A., and L.A. Wissing, Copenhagen: UNICEF.

Mondlane, R.P., A.M.P. de Graca, and G.J. Ebrahim. 1989. Skin-to-skin contact as a method of body warmth for infants of low birth weight. *Journal Tropical Pediatrics,* 35, pp. 321–26.

Neonatal Intensive Care Team. 1990. *Kangaroo Care* (brochure for parents of NICU infants). Available from Cindy Sagmeister, M.S., Neonatal Nurse Practitioner, Neonatal Intensive Care Unit, Children's Hospital, St. Paul, MN 55102.

Newport, M.A. 1984. Conserving thermal energy and social integrity in the newborn. *Western Journal of Nursing Research* 6, pp. 175–90.

Nijhuis, T. and L. Prechtl, 1982. State cycles in premature infants. *Early Human Development* (April), pp. 77–95.

Odent, S. 1983. *Birth Reborn.* New York: Random House.

Oehler, S. 1983. Sensory processing abilities of the premature infant. *Journal of The California Perinatal Association* 3(1), pp. 55–63.

Orenstein, S.R., and P.F. Whitington. 1983. Positioning for prevention of gastroesophageal reflux. *Journal of Pediatrics* 103, pp. 534–37.

Paton, J., B. Fajardo, M. Browning, and D. Fisher. 1987. Emergence of state regulation in very low birth-weight premature infants. *Pediatric Research* 21(4), p. 183A.

Pohlman, S., and C. Beardslee. 1987. Contacts experienced by neonates in intensive care environments. *Maternal-Child Nursing Journal* 16, pp. 207–26.

Powley, M., P. Nye, and P. Buckfield. 1980. Nursing jaundiced babies on lambskin. *The Lancet* 1, p. 979.

Pridham, K.F., S. Sondel, A. Chang, and C. Green. 1993. Nipple feeding for preterm infants with bronchopulmonary dysplasia. *Journal of Obstetric Gynecologic and Neonatal Nursing,* Vol. 22(2), pp. 147–58.

Purcell-Jones, G., E. Dorman, and E. Summer. 1987. The use of opiods in neonates: A retrospective study of 933 cases. *Anesthesia* 42, pp. 1316–20.

# References

Rey, E.S. and H.G. Martínez, 1983. Manejo rational de nino prematuro. *Proceedings of the Conference of 1st Curso de medicina fetal y Neonatal,* Bogota, Colombia, pp. 137–451. Manuscript available in English from UNICEF, 3 UN Plaza, New York, NY 10017.

Saunders, R.B., C.B. Friedman, and P.R. Stramoski. 1991. Feeding preterm infants: Schedule or demand? *Journal Obstetric, Gynecologic, and Neonatal Nursing* 20(3), pp. 212–18.

Schmidt, E., and G. Wittreich. 1986. Care of the abnormal newborn: A random controlled trial study of the "Kangaroo-method of care for low-birth-weight newborns." Paper presented at the Euro Amro Symposium on Appropriate Technology Following Birth, October 1986, Trieste, Italy. Unpublished manuscript available from Dr. Eberhard Schmidt, Professor of Pediatrics, University of Dusseldorf, Dusseldorf, Germany.

Scott, S. and M. Richards. 1979. Nursing low birth-weight babies on lambswool. *The Lancet,* Vol. 1, p. 1028.

Scott, S. and M. Richards. 1981. Lambswool is safer for babies. *The Lancet,* Vol. 3, March 7, 1981, p. 556.

Scott, S., T. Cole, P. Lucas, and M. Richards. 1983. Weight gain and movement patterns of very low birthweight babies nursed on lambswool. *The Lancet,* October 29, 1983, pps. 1014–16.

Sims, C.I. 1988. Kangaroo Care. *Mothering* 49 (fall), pp. 64–69.

Sleath, K. 1985. Lessons from Colombia. *Nursing Mirror* 160(4), pp. 14–16.

Sleath, K., and A. Whitelaw. 1987. Skin-to-skin contact for very low birthweight babies. In Anderson, G.C., (moderator) Natural and self-regulatory experiences postbirth: An alternative model for fullterm and premature infants. Symposium presented at the International Nursing Research Conference, Council of Nurse Researchers, October 1987, Washington, D.C.

Stennert, E., E.J. Schulte, and M. Vollrath. 1977. Incubator noise and hearing loss. *Early Human Development* I(1), pp. 113–15.

Strauch, E., S. Brandt, and J. Edwards-Beckett. 1993. Implementation of a quiet hour. Effect on noise levels and infant sleep states. *Neonatal Network* 12(2), pp. 31–35.

Thomas, K.A. 1989. How the NICU environment sounds to a preterm infant. *Maternal-Child Nursing* 14, pp. 249–51.

Tuomikoski-Koiranen, P. 1988. Kenguruhoidosts osana keskoster hoitoa ja turun yliopistollisen keskussairaalan. Unpublished manuscript available in English from Anna Maria Laiha,

University Central Hospital of Turku, Dept. of Pediatrics, 20520 Turku 52 Finland.

————. 1990. *Kangaroo Care*. Paper presented at the Third Biennial International Conference of Maternity Nurse Researchers, June 19–21, 1990, Nordic School for Public Health, Gothenberg, Sweden.

Tyler, R.M., J. Dammerks, and C. Van de Linden. 1981. Babies eat "sheepskins." *The Lancet,* January 24, 1981, p. 211.

Tynan, D.W. 1986. Behavioral stability predicts morbidity and mortality in infants from a neonatal intensive care unit. *Infant Behavior and Development* 9, pp. 71–79.

UNICEF. 1984. Kangaroo treatment saves underweight babies. News Feature, May 1984.

Updike, C., et al. 1986. Positional support for premature infants. *American Journal of Occupational Therapy* 40, pp. 712–15.

US Dept. of Health and Human Services, PHS. Monthly Vital Statistics Report. Vol. 40, No. 8(S), December 12, 1991.

————. Advance Report of Final Natality Statistics. 1989.

Virgin, C. 1987. The "Kangaroo Method" brings the child back to its mother. *Sygeplejersken* 19, pp. 10–18. English translation available from Cecilia Virgin, Abrinke 267, DK 283 Virum, Denmark.

Wahlberg, V. 1988. Alternative care for premature infants. The "Kangaroo Method." Advantages, risks, and ethical questions. *Neonatologica* 4, pp. 362–67.

Wahlberg, V., D. Affonso, and B. Persson. 1990. Kangaroo method: Alternative to premature care. Manuscript submitted for publication.

————. 1992. A retrospective comparative study using the Kangaroo method as a complement to standard incubator care. *European Journal of Public Health.* 2(1), pp. 34–37.

Wallace, J. 1991. Report presented at meeting of International Council of Nurse Researchers, November 12, 1991, Los Angeles.

Wallace, J., and J. Ridpath-Parker. 1933. Kangaroo care. *Quality management in Health Care.*

Weaver, K.A., and G.C.D. Anderson. 1988. Relationship between integrated sucking pressures and first bottle-feeding scores in premature infants. *J. Obstetric, Gynceologic and Neonatal Nursing,* 17, pp. 113–20.

Weibley, T. 1989. Inside the Incubator. *Maternal-Child Nursing* 14, pp. 96–100.

Whitelaw, A. 1986. Skin-to-skin contact in the care of the very low birthweight babies. *Maternal-Child Health* 7, pp. 242–46.

————. 1990. Kangaroo baby care: Just a nice experience or an important advance for preterm infants? *Pediatrics* 85, pp. 604–5.

Whitelaw, A., and K. Sleath. 1985. Myth of marsupial mother: Home care of very low birthweight babies in Bogota, Colombia. *The Lancet*, 1, pp. 1206–08.

Whitelaw, A., G. Heisterkamp, K. Sleath, D. Acolet, and M. Richards. 1988. Skin-to-skin contact for very low birthweight infants and their mothers: A randomized trial of "Kangaroo Care." *Archives of Diseases in Childhood* 63, pp. 1377–81.

World Health Organization. 1985. Preliminary report of joint consultation. Bogota. (Written by Bellman, et al.)

Zahr, L. 1993. Efficacy of noise control on physiology and behavior of preterm infants. Manuscript submitted for publication.

The following research investigations of Kangaroo Care are reported in the 1990 UNICEF publication entitled *First International Conference on Mother Kangaroo Program,* available free of cost from UNICEF.

1. Martínez, H., E. Rey, L. Navarrete, C.M. Marquette. Mother Kangaroo program at the Maternal-Infant Institute in Bogota, Colombia. pp. 21–44.

2. Riano de Otalora, E.M.R. Promotion, diagnosis and early intervention for sensory motor alterations in biologically high risk infants. pp. 45–56.

3. Gonzales de Pinzon, L.E. Visual and occular validation of the mother kangaroo program at the Maternal-Infant Institute in Bogota. pp. 63–86.

4. Correa, J.A., and H. Ramirez. Mother kangaroo program at the Leon the 8th Clinic neonatal service as the Social Security Hospital in Antioquia, Colombia. pp. 63–86.

5. Valencia, M.L., and J.D. Velez. Mother kangaroo program at the San Rafael Yolombo Hospital in Antioquia, Colombia. pp. 87–90.

6. Gomez, L.A. Evaluation of two years of mother kangaroo program at the Caldas Regional Hospital in Antioquia, Colombia. pp. 91–102.

7. Restrepo, F., and L.S. Lopez. Mother Kangaroo program at the General Hospital of Medellin, Colombia. pp. 103–6.
8. Gaviria, M. Mother kangaroo program, Evaluation and implementation at the San Juan de Turbo Hospital in Antioquia, Colombia. pp. 107–26.
9. Vargas, N.B., and J.F. Correa. Fathers kangarooing and their ideas and psychological responses. pp. 127–32.
10. Lopez, J.M. Experiences with the mother kangaroo method at the Joaquin Paz Borrero Hospital in Cali, Colombia. pp. 133–42.
11. Currea, S. Ambulatory care of premate infants. pp. 143–52.
12. Feraudy, P.Y. Mother kangaroo programs: Ambulatory care of the low birthweight newborn at the San Gabriel Hospital in La Paz, Bolivia. pp. 153–76.
13. Arandia, R., L. Morales. Mother kangaroo at the University of San Simeon in Cochabamba, Bolivia. pp. 177–200.
14. Camacho, L.L. Ambulatory care of premature infants in the Maternity Hospital in Quito, Ecuador. pp. 201–4.
15. Stern, C., N.L. Sloan, and E. Pinto. Mother kangaroo program—care of low birthweight neonates in Quito, Ecuador, pp. 205–32.
16. Arestegui, R.U. Evaluation of the pilot program of mother kangaroo at the San Bartolome Hospital in Lima, Peru. pp. 233–48.
17. Arestegui, R.U. Information about the mother kangaroo pilot program at the San Bartolome Hospital in Lima, Peru. pp. 249–54.
18. Martinez, J.C. Mother kangaroo program is a great opportunity for modern neonatal help. pp. 255–60.
19. Picon, C. Low birthweight premature infants: An environmental technology appropriate for resistance. pp. 261–78.
20. de Molina, H. Evaluation of mother kangaroo program at the Dr. Luis Edmundo Vasquez Hospital in Chalatenango, El Salvador. pp. 279–82.
21. Rosello, J.L.D., P.M. Lozano, and S.M. Tenzer. Impaired growth of low birthweight infants in an early discharge program. pp. 283–306.
22. Meza, G.C., J.M. Rosales, and D.P. Pineda. Efficacy of mother kangaroo program in the development of low birthweight infants at Roosevelt Hospital in Guatemala. pp. 307–50.

23. Mulet, R.C., R. Figueroa de Leon, and J. V. Gonzales. Efficacy of mother kangaroo program in the development of low birthweight neonates at the Social Security Obstetric Hospital in Guatemala. pp. 351–64.
24. de Leeuw, R. History of kangaroo care in the neonatal department of the academic medical center. pp. 365–70.
25. Davanzo, R. Care of low birthweight infants with the kangaroo mother method in developing countries. pp. 451–72.
26. Virgin, C. The "kangaroo method" brings the child back to its mother. Present and future in Denmark. pp. 475–85.

# Index

# About the Authors

Dr. Susan M. Ludington-Hoe received her Ph.D. from Texas Women's University, majoring in maternal-child health and minoring in child development. She is also a certified nurse-midwife.

Since 1976, Dr. Ludington-Hoe has published numerous scholarly articles documenting her research studies in the field of infant development, infant stimulation, and Kangaroo Care. She is also the co-author with Susan K. Golant of the popular book, *How to Have a Smarter Baby.*

Dr. Ludington-Hoe has been investigating Kangaroo Care since 1987 and to date has completed twelve research studies in this field with the support of the University of California, Los Angeles, School of Nursing, where she is currently an Associate Professor of Maternal-Child Health. She has received many grants to further her work and in 1991 was awarded a National Institutes of Health-National Center for Nursing Research grant to determine the benefits of Kangaroo Care to premature infants in the United States. To date, Dr. Ludington-Hoe and her research team have studied Kangaroo Care with over two hundred babies and their families in the United States and Central and South America.

Susan K. Golant, M.A., a writer specializing in parenting, health, and women's issues, is the author or coauthor of numerous books including *How to Have a Smarter Baby; No More Hysterectomies; Disciplining Your Preschooler and Feeling Good*

*About It; Kindergarten: It Isn't What It Used to Be; Getting Through to Your Kids; The Joys and Challenges of Raising a Gifted Child; Hardball for Women: Winning at the Game of Business; Finding Time for Fathering; 50 Ways to Keep Your Child Safe;* and *Taking Charge: Overcoming the Eight Fears of Chronic Illness.*

Her feature articles on parenting, women's issues, health, and psychology have appeared extensively in the *Los Angeles Times,* and also in such publications as *Harper's Bazaar, New Age Magazine, The Los Angeles Times Magazine, Writer's Digest, The Chicago Tribune, The Boston Globe, The Miami Herald, The Denver Post, L.A. Parent, L.A. Weekly,* and *PTA Today.*

Susan Golant lives with her husband in Los Angeles, California. She holds a master's degree in French literature and is the mother of two college-age daughters.